WORLD WAR C

WORLD WAR C

LESSONS FROM THE COVID-19 PANDEMIC
AND HOW TO PREPARE FOR THE NEXT ONE

SANJAY GUPTA, MD
WITH KRISTIN LOBERG

THORNDIKE PRESS
A part of Gale, a Cengage Company

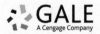

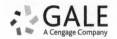

Thorndike Press® Large Print History Fact and Fiction.
The text of this Large Print edition is unabridged.
Other aspects of the book may vary from the original edition.
Set in 16 pt. Plantin.

LIBRARY OF CONGRESS CIP DATA ON FILE.
CATALOGUING IN PUBLICATION FOR THIS BOOK
IS AVAILABLE FROM THE LIBRARY OF CONGRESS.

ISBN-13: 978-1-4328-9657-7 (hardcover alk. paper)

Published in 2022 by arrangement with Simon & Schuster, Inc.

Printed in Mexico
Print Number: 01   Print Year: 2022

To the soldiers of COVID-19, from all the doctors, scientists, and health care workers, to the survivors and victims young and old.

To the children who will go bravely forward and carry these important lessons to the next generation.

And to the collective breath of the world's inhabitants . . . and the nature in which we coexist on this planet and persevere in our survival.

CONTENTS

Ingenuity, knowledge, and organization alter but cannot cancel humanity's vulnerability to invasion by parasitic forms of life. Infectious disease which antedated the emergence of humankind will last as long as humanity itself, and will surely remain, as it has been hitherto, one of the fundamental parameters and determinants of human history.

— William H. McNeill,
*Plagues and People*s (1976)

INTRODUCTION:
A "PNEUMONIA OF
UNKNOWN ORIGIN"

> The single biggest threat to man's contin-
> ued dominance on this planet is the virus.
> — Nobel Prize–winning biologist
> Joshua Lederberg (1958)

New Year's Eve 2019, Belize
I was drinking wine with, of all people,
Francis Ford Coppola while enjoying the
beautiful coast of this Central American
paradise hours before we'd ring in 2020. We
were there as part of a climate change char-
ity and had spent the day touring the surrounding coral reefs. It was a perfect day,
and I remember feeling very much at peace.
I distinctly recall Coppola asking me about
a potential new virus that had been detected
in the People's Republic of China. Earlier
that day we had both read reports buried in
the back of the newspaper about "an outbreak of respiratory illness in the central
city of Wuhan."[1] Some were already com-

11

paring it to the 2002–2003 severe acute respiratory syndrome (SARS) epidemic. The local health authority there had released a concerning epidemiological alert, stating that twenty-seven people had fallen ill with a strain of viral pneumonia, and seven were in serious condition. Fifty-nine more suspected cases with fever and dry cough were transferred to a designated hospital. While details from the Chinese government were vague, scientists and others were sounding louder and more detailed alarms. Hong Kong scientist Dr. Li-Meng Yan said a scientist at China's Center(s) for Disease Control and Prevention, with first-hand knowledge of the cases, was very worried, confidentially telling her the illness might already be spreading human-to-human. It was hard to know what to believe.

I remember everything about the moment sitting with the legendary filmmaker — the Godfather himself. I can still see both of his hands on the glass, filled with rich red wine. I can hear the clusters of family members romping on the beach and the kids giggling in the water. If I close my eyes, I can still smell the fragrant oceanfront air, rife with the tropics and the salt. Fact is, we were happy, and we were content. And, we had no idea how quickly that was all going to change.

We had no way of predicting that within just a few months, millions of people around the world would become infected, overwhelming entire health care systems. Or that many people would die alone, isolated from their family in their last moments due to the remarkable contagiousness of the virus. I could not imagine the nightmares I would continue to have of those particular scenes more than a year later. My sleeping mind filled with patients lying prone on their bellies while brave nurses in full protective moon suits held screens in front of their faces so they could try for that final goodbye.

Borders would close. Schools and colleges would shut their doors. Students would be abruptly sent home. I would spend more time with my wife and three daughters in one year than in the previous ten. Parents would wring their hands in the sudden messy juggle of overseeing their kids' distance learning and holding on to their jobs — if they were lucky enough to keep them. Stadiums, theaters, museums, playhouses, and concert halls would become desolate as professional sports and arts would suddenly cease. Businesses halted, some forever, and global economies shuddered. Large gatherings would become a distant memory. Soap, wipes, hand sanitizer, and, inexplicably, toilet paper would vanish from store shelves.

Personal protective equipment (PPE) would become as precious as gold, prompting some hospital heads to use their personal credit cards to buy whatever they could, no matter the price.[2] People would hastily write their wills, sew masks from cloth, and draw down their savings accounts. Some would tap retirement accounts.

Grandparents would soon become the loneliest members of our whole society.

Peaceful protests juxtaposed with historic civil unrest would take to the streets as the pandemic yanked the veil off deeply rooted racial injustices. Political divides would widen. Individuals who'd never contemplated buying a gun now had second thoughts. Dangerous conspiracy theories would spread as fast as the virus itself, challenging the veracity of science and the integrity of scientists. Some of those scientists would receive credible death threats, and would be forced to live with around-the-clock protection.

As dark as it was, there were also stunning bursts of light. The race for a cure would destroy academic silos. Business rivals in pharma would suddenly collaborate to develop vaccines. Public health experts, too often sidelined, would be in unprecedented high demand and quickly thrust to the front lines. Health workers everywhere would leave their families every day to be the only family of the dying, often risking their lives to do so. I still get goose bumps when I reflect on their sacrifice.

No, we didn't know the pandemic of our lifetime was already forming and gaining strength a world away as Coppola and I enjoyed that pleasant, peaceful New Year's Eve. We joked that the story unfolding might be something Coppola could put his own spin on, like some modern-era version of *Apocalypse Now.* But neither of us believed anything like that would really happen.

"In the beginning, you just never know with these things," I remember telling him somewhat nonchalantly at the time.

We also talked about another movie that might have foretold the year we were about to endure. In 2011 I had a small role playing myself in the blockbuster thriller *Contagion.* (That's the one where Gwyneth Paltrow's character brings a new pathogen home to Minnesota from Hong Kong, has a grand mal seizure in the kitchen, and ends up dying horrifically in the hospital.) I recently revisited the script of my scene with the fictional head of the CDC, Dr. Ellis Cheever (played by the great Laurence Fishburne), and was struck at how prophetic the filmmakers really were.

Me: There are stories circulating on the Internet that in India and elsewhere the drug Ribavirin has been shown to be effective against this virus. Yet the Department of Homeland Security is telling the CDC not to make any announcements until stockpiles of the drug can be secured.

Dr. Ellis Cheever: Well, Dr. Gupta, there continue to be evaluations of several drugs. Ribavirin is among them. But right now, our best defense has been social distancing. No handshaking, staying home when you're sick, washing your hands frequently.

Sound familiar? The buzz about hydroxychloroquine early on during the pandemic — and the politics swirling around its messaging — eerily parallels the movie's storyline. And Dr. Cheever's remarks about social distancing, handshaking, staying at home, and washing hands became a part of the world's daily dialogue. It was as if the writers had some access to an oracle, but the truth is it was a deep-rooted knowledge of science. Dr. Cheever's character even mentioned how difficult it was to know the actual death count, as well as the trouble with having "fifty different states . . . which means there are fifty different health departments followed by fifty different protocols." The night before filming began, the screenwriter, Scott Z. Burns, and director Steven Soderbergh had dinner with me to talk about their sci-fi movie, which they said was based on existing public health models readily available all over the world.

There is no doubt we had all sorts of warnings, and even Hollywood movies, to raise the alarms of what might be coming. The models used for *Contagion* accurately predicted that a novel virus would momentarily become the top cause of death in the United States, ahead of heart disease, cancer, and strokes. That it would bring down life expectancy a full year in the United States and at the same time lay bare the tremendous disparity in our health care system as the Latinx community lost two years of life and Blacks lost nearly three.[3]

It is hard to fathom that a microscopic blob of genetic material with no brain, eyes, ears, limbs, wings, heart, or emotions could inflict more harm than armies of soldiers in the midst of massive conflict. But SARS-CoV-2, the name of the new coronavirus that causes the wide-ranging disease named COVID-19, did just that, arriving like an alien invader and declaring war on planet Earth.

While most wars start with a declaration of sorts, World War C had a blurry, undefined, clumsy whisper of a beginning that will probably be debated for decades. We don't yet know exactly when or how this particular contagion of likely bat origin jumped into human circulation and gained such unprecedented power, speed, and virulence. What we do know is that by January 5, authorities in China and neighboring countries were publicly worried. They raised the health threat alert to Level III (Serious) in the face of a "pneumonia of unknown origin."[4] We'd all eventually find out that the disease was caused by a coronavirus, a type that belongs to a family of viruses known to cause a variety of respiratory, gastrointestinal, and neurological diseases.

A story I learned early on and that remained buried in the medical literature also happened that same January day. A sixty-one-year-old woman living in Wuhan had developed fever with chills, sore throat, and headache; she visited a local health facility for help and was given some medication that probably had no real effect on her fomenting illness.[5] Despite that, a few days later, on January 8, she took a direct flight to Bangkok, Thailand, from Wuhan City with five family members as part of a tour group going there to celebrate the Lunar New Year. I can tell you from personal experience, Bangkok's Suvarnabhumi Airport has one of the best surveillance systems in the world for detecting sick travelers to their country, so it was no surprise that her fever was immediately flagged and she was taken to a hospital. It was at that point she was found to be infected with the novel coronavirus. Although it was initially thought she was among the first people to unknowingly export the virus outside of China, newer reports show that people in the United States had already been infected by then, and likely weeks previously. In other words, the new coronavirus was infecting Americans long before the world knew it was causing a deadly outbreak in Wuhan.[6]

Let me pause here to consider the following: If you or I had flown on that same day to any major airport in the United States with flu-like symptoms, chances are that nobody at the arrival gate would've even blinked, let alone taken our temperature, or asked any questions. It was very different in many Asian countries, where they have been dealing with the threat of aberrant new viruses (with pandemic potential) for much longer than we have. The SARS outbreak nearly two decades ago was in many ways a frightening sneak preview — as well as their incentive to implement very strict public health measures.

Interestingly, the sixty-one-year-old sick woman regularly visited local markets in Wuhan before falling ill, but had not been to the Huanan Seafood Market, which was being described as the origin of the outbreak. Her case instigated international tensions between the two countries as it forced China to disclose to the world it had a problem. Once Thailand had isolated the patient, taken samples of the virus, and identified its genomics, Bangkok called Beijing and put pressure on China to confess their secret, *or else.* China initially refused, instead demanding their sick citizen back — as well as the genome sequence that Thailand now possessed. The exchange, which I learned about through an epidemiologist friend of mine who demanded strict anonymity, went something like this:

Thailand: You have a problem you have to tell the world. We're going to release the genome sequence and publish it unless you do.

Beijing: She's ours. Give her back to us — and the sequence.

Thailand: Fuck you.

By the time the United States seriously clamped down on incoming passengers from China on February 2, hundreds of thousands of people had already traveled from China to the United States, and millions more around the world. We watched as China locked down domestic travel at the end of January but left foreign travel open. While this strategy may have reduced the spread of the coronavirus within China, it did nothing to curb the viral explosion worldwide.

In a January 28 top secret intelligence briefing, national security adviser Robert O'Brien gave President Donald Trump a "jarring" warning about the virus, telling him that it would be the "biggest national security threat" of his presidency.[7] He also told Trump that it could be as bad as the influenza pandemic of 1918, which had infected half a billion people and killed an estimated 50 to 100 million worldwide, including 675,000 Americans. It was also the first time the administration was alerted to a critical detail: the possibility of asymptomatic spread. That is, many of the people transmitting the virus appeared to have no symptoms, and thus no clue they were infected.

Despite that, the initial response in our country was still based on influenza modeling, where people are considered sick only when they show symptoms. That would prove to be one of the most disastrous mistakes of the whole pandemic. In other words, even as we started to respond to the outbreak, we were essentially treating the wrong disease. At the time we were reporting cases of a few dozen sick people, there were probably already thousands of symptom-free people unwittingly spreading the virus as Americans went about their normal lives.

Most of the news stories were filled with the impeachment trial and Kobe Bryant's shocking death in a helicopter crash outside Los Angeles. It was only after the first US case of human-to-human transmission on home turf was confirmed on January 30 that the White House took more decisive action, issuing a Level 4 travel advisory for all of China and declaring a "public health emergency" the next day.[8] A Level 4 advisory is the highest advisory level, indicating a greater likelihood of life-threatening risks. The message was now clear: "Do Not Travel" to that country or leave as soon as it is safe to do so. Even then, public health experts were split about the effectiveness of restricting air travel. While they had spent their entire careers preparing for this very event, few of them had ever experienced anything like it for real. It was as if they were well-trained police officers hesitantly drawing their weapons for the first time.

As more information slowly trickled in, the level of anxiety in the public community started to fire up. Normally tempered experts increasingly used uncharacteristically hyperbolic language. Harvard-trained epidemiologist Dr. Eric Feigl-Ding's first viral tweet had already gone out on January 24 and generated him an instant following: "HOLY MOTHER OF GOD — the new coronavirus is a 3.8!!! How bad is that reproductive R0 value? It is thermonuclear pandemic level bad. . . ."[9]

Like the magnitude of an earthquake on the Richter scale, the R0 (pronounced "R-naught") is a mathematical measure of a disease's reproduction rate; it's an average measure of a virus's transmissibility but can be affected by lots of factors, including local policy, population density, and even the weather. Hence, the R0 for COVID can differ across the globe and change over time. As a comparison, the R0 of measles is 12 to 18, by far the highest known to humans, and the R0 of seasonal influenza is around 0.9 to 2.1. As Dr. Feigl-Ding tweeted, the available data at the time revealed the R0 for COVID to be somewhere between 1.4 and 3.9. That meant every single person infected with COVID could spread it to up to four others. If the R value is less than 1, an epidemic quickly dies out because each infected person generates fewer than one new infection. While some criticized Feigl-Ding for his tweet, many hailed him along with several others as being the Cassandras of COVID — those who uttered the truth but were never believed.

As a medical reporter at an international news network, I knew that my globe-trotting days would be suspended as I was forced to retreat to my compact home basement to report around the clock on every aspect of the novel coronavirus — how it travels and transmits, the molecular keys it uses to gain entry into cells, and what havoc it causes once inside the human body. And when it became clear several months into the pandemic that COVID-19 was causing neurological deficits, from minor ones like temporary loss of taste and smell to more serious problems like stroke, dementia, and psychiatric disorders, my worlds of brain surgeon and medical correspondent came crashing together.

By one large study's calculation, a third of patients diagnosed with COVID-19 experienced a psychiatric or neurological illness within six months.[10] And, more than a year later, this novel coronavirus continues to surprise us. We still don't know why some people have barely any symptoms while a similar person might end up in the ICU. We aren't sure how effectively the body clears the virus and what the persistent effects might be in those infected, including children. After this pandemic is one day declared officially over, we will likely be dealing with millions of people managing COVID-related symptoms long term, patients who are known as the long-haulers.

For more than a year, I had to wake up and steel myself every day to deliver tough news to a global audience. I would've rather been talking about extraordinary advances in science and telling stories of cultures living long, happy lives. Instead, it was a continuous narrative of increasing infections, hospitalizations, and deaths. While my medical training did prepare me for the heartbreaking task of delivering awful news to patients and their families, it never gets one bit easier, even after decades of doing it. In these tough situations, whether in medicine or media, I have tried to live by a few rules. Listen as much as you talk, and when you do speak, make sure you are understood. Speak clearly, slowly, and with great empathy and humility. You have to constantly remember that your words are fundamentally changing the course of your patient's life. It is as important to explain what you don't know as it is to be clear about what you can say with certainty. There is a balance between hope and honesty. Honesty should always lead the way, full and transparent, but hope has deep value as well. Hope is not a strategy, but it's a damn good positive motivator. And finally, whether it is speaking to a patient one-on-one or trying to educate a global audience of concerned viewers, I am always reminded of a quote from the great Maya Angelou:

"People will forget what you said, people will forget what you did, but people will never forget how you made them feel."[11]

Regardless of wherever and whenever the new coronavirus came from and when (and we'll be exploring that shortly), at least one truth prevailed that no one could deny: the human race had met its first catastrophic global pandemic in the twenty-first century. And despite our twenty-first-century medicine, glitzy computer modeling, and pandemic planning, we weren't ready.

In late 2018, I penned an op-ed warning that the Big One was coming and called for new vaccine platforms to prepare for the inevitable.[12] I stated that the Big One would likely have a greater impact on humanity than anything else happening in the world. At the time, I thought it would be a rogue and never-before-seen influenza virus from a bird or pig. Flu had always worried me, and I'm not alone in that thinking. I'd already covered the earlier strains of H1N1 (swine flu) and H5N1 (avian flu) and produced a documentary about pandemic flu. Coronaviruses were also candidates, as evidenced by SARS and Middle East respiratory syndrome or MERS (both coronaviruses), but these were thought to be too lethal to also be contagious on a level that could take off as a global pandemic. The macabre truth was that if a pathogen was highly lethal, the infected often died faster than they could spread the germ. The thought of a superbad coronavirus that could be so prismatic, wily, and deadly as SARS-CoV-2 simply did not figure even in my wildest imagination, but again, it doesn't mean we couldn't still have been so much better prepared. (For simplicity's sake, I'm going to refer to the virus, SARS-CoV-2, and its resulting disease in humans, COVID-19, as "COVID" going forward. Whether we're talking about the actual virus, the infection and the disease it causes, or the pandemic in general, "COVID" fits the bill.)

In October 2019, just months before the pandemic became a cruel global reality, the Johns Hopkins Center for Health Security and the Economist Intelligence Unit released the Global Health Security Index.[13] While the report found that "no country is fully prepared to handle an epidemic or pandemic," the United States ranked highest of all 195 countries evaluated, coming in at #1 (receiving a score of 83.5 out of 100), ahead of the United Kingdom (with a score of 77.9). While it is now clear that we didn't live up to that high standing, it is also worth recognizing the countries that were ranked poorly and truly rose to the moment. New Zealand, for instance, scored a measly 54 but had only a couple thousand cases and a handful of deaths in the first nine months. In that period, by mid-September, the United States had more than 6.5 million cases and nearly 200,000 deaths. The United States is 4 percent of the world's population but suffered more than 25 percent of the world's total infections by midsummer 2020.

In December 2020, scientists helped put the COVID numbers into perspective by comparing the daily US mortality rate with other tragedies.[14] At the time, we were experiencing a September 11, 2001, level of mortality — nearly three thousand deaths *every two days.* It was as if ten Airbus 320 jetliners, each carrying 150 passengers, were falling out of the sky and crashing every day.

It was a surprising and disturbing trend. Across the world, it was the wealthiest countries that generally fared worse in this pandemic, while many poorer countries emerged relatively unscathed. This was especially true throughout the first year of the pandemic. Later in the book we'll see how some nations looked relatively good a year later, only to let their guard down and suffer a catastrophic new wave of cases and deaths. The reasons for the discrepancies, good or bad, are as much about the virus itself as they are about human behavior.

As my friend and fellow truth seeker Jamie Metzl says, "We are all one interconnected humanity who must work together to get through this crisis." I couldn't agree more. Nowhere is our interdependence and communion more tangible than with a pandemic. We made mistakes, and that's the bad news. The good news is that we now have the chance to learn from them. No matter what you think, whom you blame, what frustrations you harbor, or whom you vote for, keep an open mind as you read this book. And, if there's one thing I've learned this past year, it's humility. I have always been Mr. Fixit. It's probably the surgeon in me, and maybe the war zone reporter as well. Get in fast and solve the problem. But sometimes, the right approach is to thoughtfully collect information, synthesize, and allow yourself to be surprised. Sometimes you have to listen intently before you can best act. My wife once told me that one of the reasons my daughters don't always come to me with their problems is because they don't want me to necessarily propose solutions; they just want me to listen.

One of the most challenging things about writing a book like this is figuring out where to end the story. In many ways, we are just beginning to understand this bug's wizardry. It still remains to be seen how effective vaccines and therapeutics will be in mitigating COVID's destructive march and ushering in the normalcy we all crave. I worry about the story of the third-world and low-income places where people are likely to be vaccinated last as wealthier nations buy supplies first. The greatest impact of COVID may be not on those whom the virus directly infects but on those shattered by the collapse of economies and health and education systems. Remote corners in Africa, Asia, South America, and India may seem distant, but they are very much a part of our global health security. You will read these words more than once: An outbreak anywhere in the world is an outbreak everywhere in the world.

One thing we do know: The virus is here to stay, so we must get used to it. Vaccines will help, but they will not give us a fairytale ending. There is no on/off switch here. Another pandemic-worthy pathogen may be right around the corner, so we need to learn how to better predict, prepare, and respond. Scientists right now are surveilling hot spots in the world where they think the next new disease-inducing piece of genetic code will emerge. As I was finishing this book, Russia reported the first case of a bird flu strain, H5N8, being passed from poultry to humans.[15] Seven workers at a poultry plant became infected and recovered, and luckily the germ did not acquire mutations fast enough to spur human-to-human transmission. But what if it had? Soon thereafter, China's National Health Commission reported the world's first human case of the H10N3 bird flu in a forty-one-year-old man who recovered and again, luckily, did not transmit the germ to others.[16] What many people don't realize is that we've had a handful of close calls in our lifetimes alone. And the chances of a pandemic happening are the same at any given time. Pandemics are random, which means they don't follow a pattern. Experts who study risk perception have a term for the mistaken view that random events are patterned: the gambler's fallacy. It's "named for the tendency of many roulette players to imagine that a number is overdue because it hasn't come up all night."[17] The probability of another pandemic hasn't increased or decreased because we've just gone through COVID.

As Yogi Berra said: It's tough to make predictions, especially about the future.

One of the most important lessons we may learn is about navigating risk. Throughout this pandemic, I have been reminded that people can look at the same level of risk and respond very differently. For example, while we are still not sure what the overall mortality of COVID is, let's say it is ~0.5 percent. For a certain group of people, they may hear that number and become unquestionably worried. After all, that means a 1 out of 200 chance of dying. They are likely to take protective measures and be particularly cautious. For others, however, it means 99.5 percent in the clear; they may not bat an eye at that risk and go about their merry way. Same data, but very different behavior. There are risks to both perspectives, either being too cavalier or too cautious, which I will explain more in chapter 6.

There are reasons we're so terrible at evaluating risk in our lives, especially under the duress of uncertainty and anxiety. And when making risky decisions breaks with social norms or personal experience, the task can feel outright paralyzing. But part of winning the next WWC is gaining the tools now to put risk into the right perspective for later.

Former White House coronavirus task force coordinator Dr. Deborah Birx calculated risk every day starting at three o'clock in the morning when she woke to evaluate new data for the Trump administration's response. Her mind raced through viral transmission numbers and mitigation strategies before she brushed her teeth. Famous for her predictive prowess, Birx had a knack for seeing things well in advance of anyone else. It was certainly true for predicting surges and new outbreaks but also in more subtle ways. In one of her last to-dos in her role, Birx told me that she had scrambled to immunize all the past presidents and their spouses. She realized that they would likely be asked to attend an important gathering sometime soon: the inauguration of President Joe Biden. If they hadn't been vaccinated, they likely wouldn't have been able to attend, but she told me she was the only one who anticipated that need. Some of the details of how she got all those dignitaries vaccinated have never been shared before.

It started with Birx forecasting, as she described it — picturing all the people soon coming to Washington from all over the country and how gregarious and social those like the Bushes and Clintons would be. "This is President Clinton with comorbidities," Birx reminded me when I interviewed her after Biden had been sworn in. She had been in a panic in the weeks before the inauguration, knowing she needed at least twenty-one days to get it done so they'd have at least some protection from a shot. She was also thinking about the former First Ladies, whom she worried about "all the time." She was wise about what role they could play: "We cannot lose our institution of kindness and they are part of those marketers — they're going to be key to the healing." She was already forecasting possible vaccine hesitancy in the future and wanted willing and trusted ambassadors, like the First Ladies (and future First Gentleman).

Inauguration Day was a potential superspreader event in her mind, because the virus was everywhere. She imagined the invisible enemy waiting for new hosts in all the little holding rooms where guests would be that day. But again, there was no plan for these VIPs to be immunized. Nor was any testing plan in place to screen the thirty thousand National Guard troops who would also descend on Washington from all over the country and set up camp for security. I would have thought that vaccinating the

Who's Who would have been planned and an easy thing to accomplish, especially since two vaccines had been authorized for emergency use by then. Even I had been vaccinated at that point. But this turned out to be hard. Birx called everyone she knew as the days ticked by. When she desperately reached out to Jared Kushner, she was down to Plan F and told him so. He had a solution — a contact Birx could call who knew all the hospital CEOs. This led Birx to finding the vaccines through New York University's Langone Hospital, and the job was done in forty-eight hours. But for Birx, the whole exercise was a reminder that no one was beyond the reach of COVID and that it had left everyone unprepared for even the most obvious and predictable challenges.

While covering this pandemic, I marked my twentieth year as a medical reporter. I started at CNN in 2001, and within weeks I was reporting from New York following the 9/11 terror attacks. That fall, I broke several stories regarding the anthrax attacks, and over the next few years, I found myself reporting from Iraq, Kuwait, and Afghanistan. I wanted to tell the stories of the human spirit under the most challenging circumstances. At times, I was thrown into the story and asked to call upon my other skill set to perform brain operations in the desert, on ships in the ocean, and after natural disasters all over the world. A couple of years before I covered the devastation of Hurricane Katrina, I traveled to Sri Lanka to show the aftermath of the tsunami that claimed more than 155,000 lives in Southeast Asia. I covered the earthquake in Haiti and the tsunami in Japan. In 2014, I was the first Western reporter who traveled to Conakry, Guinea, to investigate the deadly Ebola outbreak that would soon find its way to the United States. In many ways I have been sprinting for the last two decades, but never before have I ran so fast for so long than while covering this pandemic.

Throughout 2020 and well into 2021, I repeated the same day, over and over, waking up before sunrise to sneak in a quick run before making breakfast (and waking the whole household) and then disappearing into my makeshift basement studio. My sense of time was meaningless — a month felt like a decade, and all the typical boundaries society uses to divide time just went away. There has been no line between my life and this pandemic. I think about it all the time. When I'm not thinking about it, I'm reading about it, and when I'm not reading or thinking about it, I'm dreaming about it. My wife tells me that I'm murmuring about viral replication in my sleep. (She also says that if I were not doing such work, she would shoot me up with tranquilizers and make me sleep for a week.) Other than the virus, I was mostly thinking about my girls, really wondering how a major world disaster like this might affect them long term.

As we all go through this, I realize that for our children — despite having been born when the country was in two wars, suffering through economic recessions, and being continuously bombarded with messages about climate change — this pandemic is the most significant thing that has happened to them directly. They feel an enormous burden and responsibility, one that will shape them and their choices for the rest of their lives. When I spent time with my grandparents and asked them about their childhood, they would often talk about the flu pandemic of 1918, and I saw the impact of that experience on their behavior. The same will be true here. Whether or not children are crushed by these events or emerge more resilient depends in part on all of us, and how we proceed going forward.

We are in a war, but like all other wars, they offer infinite opportunities. They allow us to notice cracks and holes in our society and give us an urgent reason to mend those broken places, confront our failures, and move forward. World War C will change how we govern, lead, interact, travel, shop, educate, worship, and work, as well as how we think, socialize, participate in the world, parent, and take care of one another. No industry, from agriculture to animal conservation, from urban design to information technology, will be spared change.

The ultimate good news is that what we learn from this pandemic will undoubtedly change all of our lives. The hope is that we will learn how to better respond as a world, as nations, and as individuals. That the pace of medical innovation will forever be accelerated, paving the way for radical revolutions in the treatment of diseases, including intractable ones such as cancer, heart disease, and Alzheimer's that claim millions more lives. And perhaps most importantly, it will remind us that we are truly interconnected and that no matter what, we all rise, or fall — together.

At this time in the history of the Earth, many infectious disease experts believe we are entering the pandemic era. While it was previously thought to be a once-in-a-century event, they now believe most of us will experience another pandemic in our lifetime. And, if that is the case, COVID may have just provided the ultimate dress rehearsal. The pandemic has been so undeniably brutal, but the experience has also equipped us with the knowledge to not only better survive the next time around, but perhaps to even thrive. The obligation is to embrace the lessons and never forget what really happened during World War C.

■ ■ ■ ■

PART 1
HUMANITY, WE
HAVE A PROBLEM

■ ■ ■ ■

CHAPTER 1
POSTMORTEM

Throughout this pandemic, when I have reflected on the hundreds of thousands of lost lives, I am deflated and breathless. One in three Americans knows someone who died from the virus.[1] I think of the untold number of COVID orphans, the children and grandchildren left behind, and wonder how they mourn. Alone. Early on, I realized there is no center of grief inside this tragedy. The virus kept us apart. We experienced our individual losses behind closed doors — closed funeral home doors, closed nursing home doors, closed hospital doors, closed front doors.[2] With an invisible enemy in the air, we've had to set aside our emotional pain. And we can't even share our suffering with one another, as we did after other national tragedies such as 9/11, Hurricane Katrina, and the Sandy Hook Elementary School shooting. Then there's the kind of grief that isn't routinely acknowledged; it's called *disenfranchised grief.* From lost time with friends, grandchildren, and older family members to missing the milestones of life, each one of us has something to mourn.

Because we can't see the grief of others, it can feel distant and abstract. Psychologists know that during times of tragedy, we empathize with those who are suffering; we're moved, and we want to help them. But if we don't have a center of grief and all we hear are the death counts rising, we can start to experience what Azim Shariff, a social psychologist at the University of British Columbia in Canada, calls *compassion fade* or *empathy fatigue.*[3] Not only is our compassion divided among all those who are suffering, but our overall amount of compassion goes down. As Shariff explained to me, "Large numbers are not good for empathy; people who are far away from us are not good for generating empathy."

Yet there are lessons to be learned from the people who have died. Olivia knew something unkind was descending on her quickly. First came the tickle in the back of her throat, then a wave of fatigue that sent her to bed early. An active and vibrant twenty-two-year-old nursing student who moonlighted as a waitress, she had been through a stressful period in early 2020 with too many competing demands. It was now the first week of February, and although the media buzzed about a mysterious outbreak from China that could spread widely in the United States, the idea that she could be infected by a potentially deadly virus never entered her mind. Olivia had not traveled lately, and the news coming from the White House quelled her fears that a life-changing pandemic was afoot. "The overall risk to the American public remains low" went the official statement from the Department of Homeland Security.[4]

Later that night, when a dry cough and fiery sore throat woke her up, accompanied by fever, a volcanic headache, chills that no blanket could quash, and a touch of nausea, she thought it was a bad cold or perhaps a case of the flu. She was strong, she was young, and she had survived cancer as a kid, so this was nothing. She couldn't taste or smell anything, but that'd happened numerous times before with colds and sinus infections. Olivia called in sick at work the next day, skipped class, and assumed she would bounce back after some rest with chicken soup and Tylenol. The registered nurse she briefly spoke with on the 24/7 telemedicine line available to her also agreed that she'd be fine and to "weather it out," reminding her to stay hydrated.

Olivia soon lost track of the hours and days as her condition rapidly deteriorated to the point she could barely breathe or make it to the bathroom. Staunchly independent, she didn't want to burden any friends to help out, which in retrospect was a good thing because that would have given the virus an opportunity to find new hosts. Olivia died alone of respiratory failure on the couch in her tidy apartment, her family in another state still struggling to reach her and unaware of the gravity of her condition. Nobody would ever know if she died of COVID; the outbreak was still silently circulating and who knows how many others died alone as she did before the nation had any idea what it was facing.

Patrick was a fit, athletic forty-one-year-old who radiated light and had established himself as a political organizer and social entrepreneur with degrees from Georgetown, Harvard, and MIT.[5] The fifth child of Cuban exiles, he'd worked in the Obama administration and was cousin to Francis Suarez, Miami's mayor. Two days before his death, Patrick had spoken at an Elizabeth Warren campaign event in Miami, where he lived. On the last day he was seen alive,

Florida announced its first confirmed COVID cases; Patrick led a prayer group in his apartment that evening and told the doorman he did not feel well.

At 1:00 a.m., March 1, he sent a text to his siblings saying something was wrong — he was gasping for breath. Paramedics found him on March 3, Super Tuesday. The autopsy ruled his cause of death as "undiagnosed hypertensive heart disease" due to an enlarged heart. His family was flummoxed, unable to make sense of it because Patrick had never been diagnosed with any heart condition. Seven months later, in October, the family finally learned that the autopsy had also uncovered acute lung injury, including bleeding in the tiny air sacs called alveoli. Such a finding reflected similar discoveries in many early COVID deaths in New York when the first wave hit.

Alina, fifty-three years old, didn't think much about her positive COVID test in June 2020. She barely felt anything — just mild fatigue, a congested nose, and small headache — and she grew antsy staying housebound in quarantine. Her two teenage kids also tested positive, but they had a little fever and took naps. A few days later, they were seemingly ready to be teens again. Her husband was also diagnosed with the illness but escaped being hospitalized and regained nearly 100 percent of his health within a month. When the family all tested negative for the virus and were cleared to resume life, Alina thought the chapter was closed, but it was only beginning for her.

Several weeks after the rest of the family fully recovered, Alina still could not perform her normal routines. Unexplained low back pain, persistent fatigue, insomnia, and crippling anxiety she'd never had before now ruled her days. A once-avid runner, Alina fought shortness of breath, chest pain, and an unusual rapid heart rate that kept her from exercising altogether. The simplest tasks took an enormous amount of physical and mental exertion from the moment she hauled herself out of bed in the morning. On some days, walking up the stairs, preparing a meal, or engaging in a conversation felt like too much. Her intestinal system rebelled too, giving her abdominal pain and surprising diarrhea despite no changes in her healthy diet. Migraines, which she had never had before, sidelined her for days.

"My brain is broken," she told her younger sister over the phone, "and it scares me." In the car, she would reach an intersection and not know what to do. In addition to the debilitating migraines, the mental fuzziness not only took Alina far away from meeting goals in her work as a paralegal, but she started to worry about cognitive decline and dementia. How could an otherwise healthy middle-aged woman suddenly have serious problems with focusing and even forming new memories?

A quick online search led her to thousands of others complaining of "brain fog" who were deemed "long-COVID" or "long-haul" patients (more technically, post-acute COVID-19 syndrome: PACS). She also learned that this strange sequence of events — going from asymptomatic to symptomatic with no end in sight — was more common than most people realized. Doctors didn't know what to make of this. And yet according to the most recent studies, fully one-third of COVID patients become long-haulers, and nearly a third of these individuals started with asymptomatic infections.[6]

Here is what doctors do know: Persistent symptoms, including brain fogginess, are not unique to COVID. They have been documented in the medical literature going back to 1889 related to the flu.[7] In a recent historical review, early reports of the "common symptom of altered cognition" surfaced during the Russian flu pandemics of

1889 and 1892, and again during the Spanish flu pandemic of 1918.[8]* With COVID, however, the biggest concern — more so than the symptoms — was the possibility they would never go away, coming to define a person's life going forward. A full year later, Alina continued to search for pieces of her former self.

You're going to meet more COVID patients in this book. They tell harrowing stories of courage, patience, optimism, and hope. They also showcase the breadth of this

* Although the flu pandemic of 1918 is often called the Spanish flu, it did not originate in Spain. Unlike other countries that participated in World War I, Spain remained neutral and its media could report news of the flu more freely. So, when nations undergoing a wartime media blackout read in-depth accounts from Spanish news sources, especially after Spain's King Alfonso XIII came down with the illness, people assumed that Spain was the pandemic's ground zero. But that was likely not the case. Scientists are still unsure of its birthplace, with Britain, France, and China all candidates. It may have even originated in the United States, where the first known case was reported at a military base in Kansas on March 11, 1918.

disease, which has affected individuals in spectacularly different and varied ways. I've spoken to identical twins who contracted the same virus as housemates but one ended up on a ventilator while the other coped relatively well. How can that be? As we'll see later on, the baffling nature of this virus that kills one person in a matter of days while leaving another unscathed is partly what makes this pandemic such an urgent mystery to solve. In the millions of lives lost, there are important lessons, and we must take the time to learn them, no matter how painful.

In medicine, it can sometimes take decades to critically dissect a new disease and fully comprehend the biology and behavior of a germ and how it affects people across the ages, sometimes disproportionately. The answers are not nearly as intuitive as you may think. With the 2009 H1N1 pandemic, those most likely to require hospitalization were under the age of ten. The thinking was that the youngest had never been exposed to anything close to this novel strain of flu and therefore had no innate immunity. With avian flu, or H5N1, those most affected were between the ages of ten and forty: It was the body's own overzealous inflammatory response that probably increased the risk of death, something more common in young adults. With COVID, though, it was the elderly who were most likely to get sick and die of this disease: 80 percent of the mortality happened in those over the age of sixty-five. But in the early days, even this simple insight had not been recognized or documented.

And that insight would later lead to confusion and deadly missteps. Thinking COVID was an "old person's disease," younger Americans were inclined to ignore the government directives, believing they would not get infected or could recover easily. As the virus mutated, however, it began to find younger and younger hosts to infect — especially once older generations gained protection through vaccination. And by spring 2021, hospitalizations of people in their twenties and thirties with COVID, some with severe symptoms, jumped. The experiences of Olivia, Patrick, and Alina show that despite the stereotype of COVID decimating those sixty-five and older, COVID has been underestimated as a virus with the power to kill people in their prime or leave those who survive with lasting symptoms. It also has the power to modify itself as it seeks to spread. That's why collecting the lessons of this pandemic will help prepare for a better, safer future. We cannot get pandemic amnesia.

CAUSE OF DEATH

Doctors often like to joke that internal medicine docs know everything — but do nothing. Surgeons know nothing — but do everything. And pathologists, well, they know everything and they do everything — but a day too late. A version of this is often attributed to serial suspense writer Robin Cook who used it in his 1983 nail-biter *Godplayer.* Cook is famous for popularizing the medical thriller genre; many of his books address topics affecting public health, and he had written plenty of infectious disease–themed novels, including *Outbreak, Contagion,* and *Pandemic.* In his books, and those of most physician authors, I have often seen another important theme emerge as well: introspection. Contrary to what most people think, I believe doctors are a lot more self-reflective than we are reputed to be.

That's partly because most doctors I know are defined by their failures far more than their successes. We are tormented at the idea of a patient dying a preventable death, and we have codified ways that force us to evaluate our mistakes, our complications — and, yes, the deaths themselves — in a formal way. Most hospitals have a regular meeting behind closed doors where we openly discuss these outcomes among ourselves. In some places the conference is called D and C (for Death and Complications) or M and M (for Morbidity and Mortality). Take it from me: It is hard to bear witness, to stand at that lectern baring your soul.

In some ways, the autopsy is the physical embodiment of these introspections. It is gruesome and emotionally devastating to watch, especially knowing the work will do nothing for the patient on the table. We conduct this postmortem so that others in the future can live and not suffer the same preventable death.

Postmortems on COVID victims have begun to reveal more about the virus's wrath in a human body — from its debris in the brain down to "COVID toes." But before we get to those details in chapter 3, there's another type of postmortem to consider first. About a year into the pandemic, after we surpassed more than half a million American deaths and Joe Biden had been sworn into office, I conducted a postmortem with six of the doctors Donald Trump had charged with leading the way out of the pandemic.[9] Of the six, many of whom were seen momentarily at the lectern in the White House briefing room, Dr. Anthony (Tony) Fauci, director of the National Institute of Allergy and Infectious Diseases (NIAID) since 1984, was the only one who made the transition to the new Biden team as the president's chief medical adviser. The others are private citizens now, unbridled and unrestrained.

Over a few weeks, in Houston, Washington, DC, and Baltimore, our team secured nondescript, large hotel ballrooms with plenty of space and ventilation to allow these extraordinary one-on-one conversations to take place in strict confidence. Given our shared medical backgrounds, I explained to each of the doctors that I was going to frame the discussions in a way that would be tough but familiar: as an autopsy. We were going to meticulously dissect and discuss how the United States became home to the worst COVID outbreak on the planet.

We are one of the richest countries in the world with a sophisticated and expensive health care system. I remember reflecting on our #1 ranking for pandemic preparedness by Johns Hopkins when I watched what was happening in Los Angeles during the 2021 winter surge of COVID cases that hit after the holidays. These were scenes I had previously witnessed only in disaster-stricken areas around the world. By mid-January, one person in L.A. was dying every six minutes, and hospitals were cracking under the strain as ambulances circled for hours trying to find emergency rooms that could take one more patient.[10] We were nearly a year into the pandemic and were still unable to stop it.

On top of that we also have the largest income inequality in the developed world and most of the developing world. This pandemic had illuminated that stark racial and economic divide. By mid-February, COVID had killed Black residents in L.A. at nearly twice the rate and Latinx at nearly three times the rate of white Angelenos.[11] Yet halfway around the world in Asia's largest slum, Mumbai's Dharavi, where a million residents live in closely packed shanties and multigenerational families share a single room, the death rate was curiously minuscule (this would soon change and shockingly so, but I'll get to that later because it's part of the story — and the lessons). Similarly, in Nigeria, with a population of some 200 million, the reported death rate was less than a hundredth of the US rate. Black and brown Americans were not only the most adversely affected in the United States; as an independent demographic, their infection and mortality rates were among the highest in the world.[12]

What struck me a year later when I sat down for more than twenty hours of these interviews with the people initially in charge of the pandemic response was the realization that their background and credentials would have led anyone to believe they were the best people for the job. We had our Avenger team in place. They may not have all agreed on what steps to take and lively, heated discussions would take place, but they respected one another's expertise and were the most qualified people to make decisions. Consider Dr. Robert Kadlec, who was appointed by President Trump in 2017 to head the Office of the Assistant Secretary for Preparedness and Response (ASPR) at the Department of Health and Human Services. Interestingly, ASPR was created by legislation and signed into law by President Bush in 2006 — just a year after Bush, while vacationing in Texas, could not put down a copy of John M. Barry's book about the 1918 flu pandemic. Detailing the mysterious plague that "would kill more people than the outbreak of any other disease in human history," Barry, a historian, scared the breath out of Bush, prompting the president to call his top Homeland Security adviser, Fran Townsend, into the Oval Office when he returned to Washington.[13] He shared his copy of *The Great Influenza* with her and said, "You've got to read this." He then added, "Look, this happens every hundred years. We need a national strategy."

Out of that conversation came our country's most comprehensive pandemic playbook. According to Townsend who publicly shared the experience with the media, the plan included diagrams for a global early-warning system; funding to develop new vaccine technologies; and a strong national stockpile of crucial emergency supplies that would be in high demand, such as protective clothing, face masks, and ventilators. Many of Bush's doubtful aides and cabinet officials balked at the efforts, which also included gaming exercises to test the ideas and protocols. But Bush insisted on the plan; one aide even described him as "obsessed" with it.[14] He set out to spend $7 billion on it, or about $10 billion in today's dollars. To Townsend, who at the time felt buried by more pressing crises such as counterterrorism, hurricanes, and wildfires, Bush said something prophetic: "It may not happen on our watch, but the nation needs the plan." He also stated a truism we've all come to learn the hard way fifteen years later: "A pandemic is a lot like a forest fire. If caught early it might be extinguished with limited damage. If allowed to smolder, undetected, it can grow to an inferno that can spread quickly beyond our ability to control it."[15] Although much of the ambitious plan was shelved in subsequent years and never fully realized, some things like the establishment of ASPR remained lying in wait for 2020.

Prior to Kadlec's role at ASPR, he'd spent his life on biodefense strategy as a physician and career officer in the US Air Force. While in the Bush administration, he had helped lead the response to 9/11, the subsequent anthrax attacks, and all the devastating hurricanes including Katrina that I covered as a reporter. Years later, Kadlec was still dealing with a hurricane, this one called Dorian and aimed at Puerto Rico, when news of a strange cluster of pneumonia patients started to surface. At first, it was background noise to his focus on Dorian's aftermath. Like me, he was somewhat nonchalant when first hearing about the strange new pneumonia on the other side of the world. He could not imagine a viral storm eclipsing the stress he had experienced after five combat tours in Iraq. But it did. "I think I have PTSD from this experience," he told me, his eyes welling up.

Adding to his feelings of despair was the sinking realization that not only was this pandemic tragic in its scope; it was also nearly entirely predictable and preventable based on a series of tabletop modeling exercises he had code-named Crimson Contagion back in 2019.[16] This simulated scenario featured a respiratory virus from China that flew around the world and was first detected in Chicago. Forty-seven days later, the World Health Organization (WHO) declared a pandemic, but by then it was too late: 110 million Americans were expected to become ill, leading to 7.7 million hospitalized and 586,000 dead. Sound familiar?

Despite Johns Hopkins's optimism, the October 2019 draft report of the exercise showed just how underfunded, underprepared, and uncoordinated the federal government would be for a life-or-death war with a new virus for which no treatment or antidote existed. The report was marked "not to be disclosed." Crimson Contagion exposed the shortcomings of our response system that eventually, and eerily, played out in reality. Most notable in the mock pandemic were the repeated instances of "confusion." Federal agencies wrestled with who was in charge. State officials and hospitals struggled to figure out what supplies were available or stockpiled. Cities and states went their own ways on school closings. The fiction would soon turn into nonfiction.

For Kadlec, the three biggest lessons learned from the experiment were that when a pandemic hits, you must know who is in charge, establish the supply chain and source materials for things like personal protective equipment (PPE) and testing kits, and find the money to pay for all the needs in the response. We will talk about leadership later, but the state of our emergency supply chain of PPE, medicines, ventilators, and other medical equipment was a complete mystery at the beginning of the pandemic. With no systems in place, we had to start from scratch. In Crimson Contagion, Kadlec and his team estimated that the United States would need $10 billion — the same number Bush had projected — in order to prepare for such an event. That money was never authorized.

Instead, in the twelve months of Kadlec's tenure at ASPR during the COVID pandemic, he spent $35 billion and got an additional $23.6 billion from Congress in December 2020 to react to the burgeoning pandemic. But those numbers didn't even touch the costs related to losing hundreds of thousands of lives, jobs, businesses, and livelihoods. To put $10 billion into perspective, it's about $30 per citizen or $3 a year for ten years, a pittance that could have made the United States pandemic proof, according to Kadlec. If the virus was a national security threat, protecting the country against it would have cost less than the price of a single aircraft carrier. We have eleven active aircraft carriers, more than any other country in the world, but authorizing some of that money to fight a potential unseen enemy was not a gamble politicians were willing to take. And as a country, we paid an enormous price for that oversight. In one of Joe Biden's first orders of business as the new president in 2021, the United States passed a COVID relief package that cost nearly $2 trillion.[17]

Had a different cast of characters been placed in leadership positions on the task force, would the outcome have been any different? No one can answer that. As I spent time with the doctors during my interviews and countless early-morning and late-night calls, another question came up repeatedly: "If you are being marginalized or even silenced, why stay in the job?"

From all of them came some version of the same answer: "I believed I was the best person for the job, and I was worried that if I left, I would be replaced with someone less effective and more political." When they realized their input was being increasingly subdued by the White House, they found ways to carry on their crusade against the pandemic. To those of us on the outside, by May 2020 it appeared that the task force had been disbanded because it no longer appeared in the media's coverage of Trump's press briefings. In fact, meetings were continuing, but behind closed doors — usually in Birx's office in person or virtually. Birx privately met with Tony Fauci, CDC director Bob Redfield, and then-FDA commissioner Stephen Hahn three or four times a week in what was called the Doctors Group. The group wasn't secret, but not many people knew about it. They talked about the medical issues that needed to be addressed and continued to analyze the pattern of the outbreak.

Dr. Birx was candid with Vice President Mike Pence, who had been her ally since she arrived and never hesitated to follow her lead. As soon as she noticed patterns that showed the ferocity of the virus's spread in mid to late summer, she went to Pence with her graphs and charts. "And when that happens with these kinds of curves," she told him, "it's going to be worse than anything we have seen before." He looked at her squarely and said, "You do what you need to do." That was permission to hit the road.

Birx used Pence's plane to go state by state, rolling her suitcase to one rental car after another to meet with people in their communities. Her travels to states turned out to be her secret for having a greater impact. On the road, she met a different tone in the people she encountered from what she'd experienced in the White House. In her words, "There was constant tension between working hard to follow the rules I was given and then working hard to make sure I could get information out that was critical to the states and American people. And it was interesting to me how that played out, and how I would be allowed to be very frank and *facilitated* to be frank with regional and local press, governors and mayors, and be very clear about mask mandates, closing bars, and severely restricting indoor dining, and all of these elements that I was never allowed to say nationally."

Most of the governors and mayors listened

to and followed her advice precisely. In one school district, for example, she urged testing all teachers with the idea that they would represent the community — not because she thought that the schools were a big spreading event. "It's why we asked every hospital to routinely test all of their staff and to triangulate that back to a zip code so you can see where the spread was occurring," she said. This kind of counter-intuitive thinking fell on deaf ears in the White House. Despite Trump's frank "this is deadly stuff" remark to journalist Bob Woodward back in the first week of February, at no time did anyone in the White House give Birx the impression that any of them thought there was significant asymptomatic spread, that the level of contagion was high, and that the disease was this deadly.[18] No wonder Birx was nicknamed Dr. Doom in the lower level of the West Wing.

For his part, Tony Fauci delivered his science-based message to every media outlet possible, from comedy shows and celebrity podcasts to *Sesame Street*. And he often told people in the White House what they didn't want to hear. At the back of his mind was a sage piece of advice he'd learned from a mentor soon after he became director of the National Institute of Allergy and Infectious Diseases under Ronald Reagan: "Do yourself a favor, Tony. Every time you go into the White House, whisper to yourself *This may be the last time I'm walking into the White House.*" Fauci wasn't someone who'd fall prey to the president's reality distortion field — a term used to describe the unique, often illusionary environment that surrounds an individual in power where sycophants abound, and it can be hard to tell that leader the truth if it goes against their wishes or ideology.[19] Fauci stuck to his personal constitution of following the facts, even at the risk of getting ousted by Trump. Resisting the gravitational pull of the White House and Oval Office in particular is a job unto itself.

Politics got in the way for sure, but a tragedy of this magnitude doesn't have a single cause. The doctors were in agreement about an outrageous reality: The vast majority of deaths in the United States could have been avoided. At the end of my interview with Kadlec, he looked at me and said, "Hubris. Hubris was the cause of death in this autopsy."

When faced with the unknown, we like to turn away and unsee whatever makes us uncomfortable and afraid. Pandemic denialism is hardly new. In *A Journal of the Plague Year,* Daniel Defoe wrote that in 1665, municipal authorities in London initially refused to accept that anything unusual was happening, then tried to shield information from the public, until the spike in deaths made it impossible to deny the fearsome bubonic plague. By that point, all the authorities could do was lock victims and their families in their homes in a futile attempt to stop the spread. In the book's opening pages, Defoe's words reveal the main differences between the plague of his era and ours: "It mattered not from whence it came. . . . We had no such thing as printed newspapers in those days to spread rumors and reports of things."[20]

Defoe was referring to the fact that authorities knew the scourge was making another death-reaping round, what would be London's last epidemic of bubonic plague, but they could keep it secret because there was no way to correspond with people easily through the kind of media system we have today, more than 350 years later. The reality of COVID's spread could not be covered up as people shared the savagery of the illness through media, with an important caveat: Although we have plenty of publications and broadcast media to tell us what's going on, these vehicles also have the capacity to circulate false ideas and disinformation.

Like the London authorities trying to conceal the plague's entrance into the city, we similarly experienced division, dysfunction, and lack of truth telling among our leaders as this twenty-first-century plague took off. I can only imagine how the Great Plague of London, which claimed nearly a quarter of the population, would have played out with modern technology and savvy modes of communication. Defoe's book, which was published fifty-seven years after the year-long event, was intended to be a forewarning as well as a practical handbook of what to do and, more importantly, what to avoid during a deadly outbreak, should one happen again. Defoe's primary source of data for his story was the Bills of Mortality — the one-page weekly reports that documented who died and from what. These pages served as leaflets, or handbills, that were posted in public places to alert people that the plague was spreading. It was the only way to disseminate the news. For Defoe, the collection of mortality bills was his way of charting the course of the Black Death's rise and fall throughout 1665,* peaking in the hot summer and declining by Christmas. By most measures, the Bills of Mortality offered the first records in the world of the spread of a disease; it was also the first time in human history that a pattern was reflected in the data: You could see the plague take off, kill increasingly more people on a weekly basis, and then retreat.

Today our disease- and death-tracking methods are more sophisticated, but they are equally revealing and instructive. On page 37 is a journal of our plague year from the first week of March 2020 to a full year later.

Within the data and the graphs of trajectories like this one lie so many stories, insights, and lessons. It's amazing to see such discrepancies among countries, each of which

* The Bills of Mortality in the collection that Defoe used for his book were dated from December 27, 1664, through December 19, 1665. Serial entrepreneur and inventor Jay Walker owns a leather-bound and vellum-paged volume of the original bills in his private Library of the History of Human Imagination in Connecticut.

followed its own pandemic response proto-
col with various forms of mitigation strategies and lockdowns. Most remarkable is the
difference between wealthy and poor nations, but in nearly the opposite way we
have come to expect. While infectious
disease outbreaks typically crush poorer
countries, this novel coronavirus disproportionately devastated many of the world's
wealthiest nations. Why? The path of the
disease worldwide also took wild and unpre-
dictable lurches in one direction and then
another.

*Daily New Confirmed COVID-19 Cases Per
Million People*

At the beginning of March 2020, for
instance, South Korea was averaging more
than 550 new daily confirmed cases, compared with just 53 in the United Kingdom,
which has a similar population size.[22] At
the end of the month, however, South
Korea had 125; the United Kingdom was at
4,500 and climbing while simultaneously
struggling to establish basic systems for supplies, testing, and contact tracing. South
Korea may not have had as robust of a
health care system as the United Kingdom,
but it had a robust public health strategy
executed early and strongly to gain control

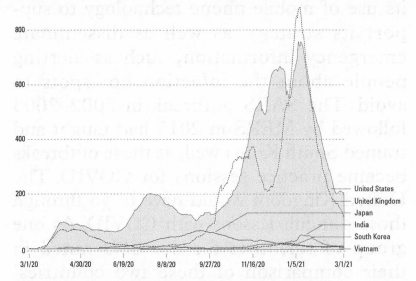

800	
600	
400	United States
200	United Kingdom
	Japan
	India
	South Korea
0	Vietnam

3/1/20 4/30/20 6/19/20 8/8/20 9/27/20 11/16/20 1/5/21 3/1/21

Shown is the rolling seven-day average. The number of confirmed cases is lower than the number of actual cases; the main reason for that is limited testing.
Source: Johns Hopkins University CSSE COVID-19 Data[21]

of the virus's spread. The key difference was that South Korea rapidly adopted a "test, trace, isolate, and treat" plan of action, whereby people with suspected disease were tested, their contacts were identified, strict isolation was enforced, and free treatment was provided to those infected, with compensation for people who had to self-isolate. This did not happen in the United Kingdom, where testing was limited early on and then both contact tracing and community monitoring were abandoned in March. South Korea was also sprinting ahead with

71

its use of mobile phone technology to support its strategy, as well as disseminate emergency information, such as alerting people about the infection hot spots to avoid. The SARS outbreak in 2002–2003 followed by MERS in 2015 had taught and trained South Korea well, as those outbreaks became practice sessions for COVID. The United Kingdom would have to go through those difficult lessons with COVID. As one group of scientists for the *BMJ* noted in their comparison of these two countries' responses, "South Korea was quicker to base decisions on the precautionary principle when the evidence was unclear," whereas the United Kingdom relied heavily on mathematical models and adopted policy led by science that arrived too late.[23] In other words, South Korea approached the problem assuming the worst-case scenario, while the United Kingdom depended on knowledge that was outdated.

Former CDC director Bob Redfield thinks the general unhealthiness of the American people also played a big role in our tragic death count. It didn't help, he says, that we went into this war unfit, with chronic conditions like obesity, diabetes, kidney disease, and cardiovascular disorders, among others — all of which alone demand a lot of attention from our body. These are mostly diseases of privilege — of wealthy nations. We are victims of our own prosperity. Although chronic, preventable diseases like obesity are on the rise throughout the world, including poorer nations, high-income countries like the United States share a much higher percentage of obesity cases worldwide. The large outliers among rich countries are Japan and South Korea, where only around 5 percent of premature deaths are attributed to obesity (as a comparison, obesity accounts for 18 percent of deaths among Americans ages forty to eight-five).[24]

Some of the poorer countries may have had another advantage as well, one that wasn't seriously considered for months into the pandemic: preexisting immunity. As we'll see, a region's history of infection can have a profound impact on the vulnerability of its inhabitants. Perhaps that helps explain why the coronavirus has not been a "Chinese flu" but rather a Western malady when you consider where the most damage was inflicted. If you want to understand why a particular nation fared poorly or did well, one of the most significant pieces of data would be where on the planet it was located.

Consider that there were close to 9,000 cases per 100,000 people in the United

States, whereas in India, it was about a tenth of that throughout the first year of the pandemic, even though Asia has some of the most population-dense areas in the world. Some European countries, for another example, took extreme measures but still went on a deadly roller-coaster ride, while others managed to gain control of the virus relatively early on and enough to look almost normal again long before the start of 2021. What explains this? What is the most effective tool for containing a virus on the loose? Do people in East Asia, a region with far fewer COVID casualties than other parts of the world, have some innate immunity from living where coronaviruses are endemic? Could they have shown up to the COVID war equipped with protective gear already? Studies are underway to explore this possibility. The pattern of the disease's gravity across the globe is not the same, and in spots where you'd think the virus would decimate a nation, such as impoverished, densely populated places where the public health infrastructure is practically nonexistent, it didn't happen. Now, there are some exceptions to this pattern that became evident after the pandemic's first year, but it's important to note that generally speaking, wealth and advanced health care systems did not necessarily give nations an advantage in controlling the virus's spread.

All the countries in East Asia, Southeast Asia, and North Asia — a diverse region with a mix of wealthy and poor nations — experienced a lower rate of the disease and death in the first year even though their health care systems, be they national health care systems or patchwork ones, were different. For example, Japan and South Korea had a much lower COVID rate and mortality than the United States or United Kingdom, even after adjusting for the differences in population sizes. Highly populated countries in that region, such as the Philippines and Indonesia, had lower COVID rates and mortality compared to developed countries such as Germany and Norway, also after adjusting for population size. The European Union performed, on average, three thousand times worse than Taiwan, where the death rate was a minuscule 0.42 per million until a slight surge in late spring of 2021. Cambodia reported only a single death and just over one thousand cases by March 2021. This was followed by a new wave of infections but the numbers still paled in comparison to the waves seen in the West throughout 2020 and early 2021.

Such an odd pattern is not new to this

pandemic. The lopsidedness of less casualties at a pandemic's origin — and graver disease in places far from the origin — has also been documented in the three main flu pandemics in the past century. While the 1918 pandemic may have originated in the United States, it took more lives on other continents, such as Asia and Europe. The 1957 and 1968 flu pandemics started in China but caused much more death in the United States and Europe. The increased aggressiveness of these pandemics in regions far from their origin cannot be fully explained by factors like underlying chronic conditions or age. We know that the highest mortality for COVID is among elderly populations, but we can't neglect the fact that Japan has the oldest population in the world and still has had a relatively low COVID death rate.

As a group of researchers from Oregon State and the University of Nevada noted, "[A] compelling explanation for the pattern might be a partial preexisting cross-immunity to these viruses in areas close to the origin of the pandemics."[25] In another published summary article, researchers from the Center for Infectious Disease and Vaccine Research at La Jolla Institute for Immunology put forth an intriguing possibility: A large percentage of the population appears to have immune cells that are able to recognize parts of the COVID virus, and that may possibly give them a head start in fighting off the infection.[26] In other words, some people may have some unknown degree of protection even without ever being exposed to COVID This might also help account for the wide range of symptoms people experienced. We'll be probing more deeply into this phenomenon so that we can better understand what this means for combating future pandemics. One thing is for certain: it casts the word *novel* under a whole new light.

NOVELTY

I've thought a lot about the significance of the word *novel* from both a biological standpoint and a cognitive, psychological one. For me, one of the greatest lessons that may come out of this pandemic is the ability to mentally process something novel and bring risk into proper perspective at the same time to inform and possibly modify behavior. After all, when was the *last* time we, as adults and as a society, truly experienced something for the *first* time? Do you remember ever being in a situation that was so unfamiliar that you had no sense of up or down?

We go through each day having millions of microexperiences, and the vast majority of them are completely expected, habituated, and contextualized. When we are surprised, we automatically put that surprise inside a box that we can understand and explain. It is human nature to look for the familiar and discard the inconsistencies. When something highly unusual or unprecedented happens in our lives, the mind is very good at eliminating those incidents. Forgetting them. Pretending they never existed. If it doesn't make sense or creates too much conflict in our own brains, it doesn't fit the narrative our minds have created to guide our lives.

When this novel coronavirus emerged, many scientists, public health officials, and doctors — myself included — immediately looked to other deadly coronaviruses, such as SARS and MERS, for clues to predict how this one would behave. It was almost a reflex. *Coronavirus from China? That belongs in the SARS box.* Or: *A burgeoning pandemic? The last pandemic I covered was H1N1 or swine flu in 2009. I will put this novel virus in that box.* But it was nothing like either of them, and the truth is that there was no standardized box in which to place

COVID I remember putting my head down deep into this, taking in all the information I could: reading research papers and unpublished preproofs; conducting Zoom calls with sources in China, South Korea, and Japan; talking to experts like Tony Fauci and global health expert Peter Daszak, whose research has been key to understanding the impact of emerging diseases.[27] And I remember that everyone had a theory about some aspect of this novel coronavirus. Even my mother had a theory.

In the earliest days, we thought human-to-human transmissibility was unlikely, that masks weren't particularly helpful, that people couldn't spread it asymptomatically or through the air. Maybe we just hoped these things would be true — magical thinking to try and convince ourselves the pandemic wasn't the black swan event we had been fearing for a hundred years. But we were wrong. In fact, our existing fund of knowledge turned out to be a major *obstacle* in our thinking — it got in our way. Just consider that. If you are dealing with something truly novel, it makes sense to bring in people from completely different walks of life because they don't immediately fall into the trap of trying to incorrectly place that novel thing into a familiar box. But we didn't do that, and instead kept looking for our comfortable boxes. It was a humbling experience for everyone, even for people like Tony Fauci, who got agitated when I reminded him that he had said, "In the history of respiratory viruses, there's never been one that has spread so efficiently asymptomatically."

When the kids got sent home from school in early March and most businesses shut their doors, people assumed the lockdown would be a few weeks, maybe a month. Easter was declared the goal for gaining our freedom and normalcy again. It was a complete fantasy in retrospect, but the alternative — the reality of a virus engulfing the globe and robbing our way of life — was not digestible. President Trump told me in late February that he didn't want to panic the American public and that "we're ready for it," which was another manifestation of ignoring a catastrophe despite clues falling from the sky. Again, I know being honest and direct and telling people the truth is sometimes hard.

Over the past few decades, I have learned that presenting a plan alongside the problem doesn't soften the blow of terrible news, but it can help mitigate the panic. People will feel less helpless and instead be driven to take action and do something. A report by Columbia University stated that had we taken action and carried out control measures like physical distancing and mask wearing just one to two weeks earlier, a substantial number of cases and deaths — more than half — could have been averted.[28] From Dr. Birx's perspective, after our initial surge in the spring, which killed about 100,000 Americans, "All of the rest of them, in my mind," she told me, "could have been mitigated or decreased substantially if we took the lessons we had learned from that moment and ensured we utilized them city by city and county by county, state by state."[29]

February 2020 has been named The Lost Month.[30] It was a crucial time, but we as a nation were not in step with the science. We may not have been masked yet, but we were blindfolded by a lack of imagination. Interestingly, when the 9/11 Commission presented its conclusions on how the attacks could have been prevented, four kinds of failures were revealed: policy, capabilities, management, and imagination.[31] These failures spectacularly repeated themselves in the pandemic. Just as we could not, prior to 9/11, ever imagine airplanes weaponized like that to mass-murder thousands of people, we could not imagine an invisible virus tramping across our turf where we have some of the best doctors and scientists in the world. When we were told on February 2 that the risk of widespread infection across America was "low," we had only about a dozen confirmed cases; within six weeks, there were nearly 3,500 confirmed. Like an echo from 9/11's failures, we similarly lapsed in policies, capabilities, and management when COVID crashed into our lives. An honest assessment of the problem and plan also sets people's expectations, which is critically important.

If I had known in January 2020 that for the next eighteen months, we'd be living in COVID lockdown life, it would have been a very difficult fact to accept, but in at least one way, it would have been easier: There would be a timetable about how things should progress — and a tangible end. The human mind prefers the certainty and finality of a countdown to zero, as opposed to the inherent ambiguity of counting up for what feels like forever. We're not nearly as good at counting up as we are at counting down.[32] However painful and long, when we count down, we still have the anticipation of an end date.

DARING TO USE THE P WORD

On March 9, 2020, I published a column on CNN's website declaring the fomenting crisis a pandemic and used that weighty term on television for the first time.[33] The reaction was swift. Some accused me of hyping the story, and serious threats directed at me were reported to CNN security and the local police. Our family never experienced danger, but every night, I quietly padded around the house after the girls were asleep to triple-check that all the doors were locked. I was glad to have dogs I knew could alert us if necessary.

Calling it a pandemic was not a decision I took lightly and it was not intended to spark fear. At the time there were more than 100,000 cases and over 3,000 deaths attributed to this new virus globally, and the numbers were climbing. The virus had found a foothold on every continent except Antarctica. Contrary to what you might think, the specific criteria for a pandemic are not universally defined, but there are three general indicators: (1) a virus that can cause illness or death, (2) sustained person-to-person transmission of that virus, and (3) evidence of spread throughout the world. The CDC says a pandemic is "an epidemic that has spread over several countries or continents, usually affecting a large number of people," while an epidemic is "an increase, often sudden, in the number of cases of a disease above what is normally expected in that population."[34] By the time CNN called it, some had already raised the alarm, including the director of the CDC's National Center for Immunization and Respiratory Diseases, Dr. Nancy Messonnier, who used the P word in a late February press conference.[35]

On February 25, as she and her team at the CDC began preparing, Messonnier went further: "It's not so much a question of if this will happen anymore but rather more a question of exactly when this will happen and how many people in this country will have severe illness." She went on to say, "I understand this whole situation may seem overwhelming and that disruption to everyday life may be severe. But these are things that people need to start thinking about now. I had a conversation with my family over breakfast this morning and I told my children that while I didn't think that they were at risk right now, we as a family need to be preparing for significant disruption of our lives. . . . I also want to acknowledge the importance of uncertainty. During an outbreak with a new virus, there is a lot of uncertainty."[36]

Those comments didn't make the Trump administration happy. From their perspective, the virus was "contained" in the United States and "very well under control."[37] Two days after Messonnier's remarks, the White House appointed Birx to the position of coronavirus response coordinator, and she became the only person on the task force to work from an office in the White House. After Dr. Messonnier's bold and honest statements, she no longer appeared at public briefings of the White House coronavirus task force.

The shift in thinking among public health officials was a turning point for me in my mind. I had a bad feeling about what we were in for — a move from the idea that we could get our arms around this (containment) to barely keeping up and just trying to slow it down (mitigation). I also had a hunch that almost no American was psychically prepared to absorb the new reality. In my "pandemic" article for CNN.com, I said things no one wanted to hear:[38]

Now is the time to prepare for what may be ahead. That could mean quarantines, closed schools and cancelled events in your town. It might mean strain at work or taking a break from hobbies that usually bring you joy. It might mean putting off a family vacation or catching up over the phone instead of getting together.

Humanity has overcome pandemics before. In this globally connected world, we may be asked to add more social distance between each other, but that doesn't mean we can't still collectively come together as a nation and as a world. This is a crisis we can overcome if we can work together.

My words were jarring for people. Many understood the gravity of the situation and started to take action. Others would go on to declare COVID a "hoax," perhaps trying to call my bluff. Whatever the reason, it was difficult to watch a country like the United States fail to execute the most basic public health strategies.

We were better at getting the big things right. We made remarkable progress in scientific and medical arenas, developing protocols and therapeutics for people who got sick. Most notable of all, we managed to develop several vaccines at historic speed. Vaccines are one of the greatest technological innovations in human history, and once again, as with smallpox, polio, and dozens of other vaccines, they would eventually rescue us, but they can never work as quickly as changes in human behavior.

Public health experts had given us the warnings and the tools, however basic, throughout this pandemic: physically distance, wear a face mask, wash our hands often. Other countries, such as South Korea, where the first patient was diagnosed the same day the first US patient was diagnosed, leaned into those basic public health measures and have done exponentially better. Their death count has been in the low thousands. Ours: in the hundreds of thousands — more than half a million.

So if I had to answer the question about primary cause of death here, I'd call it multisystem organ failure, ranging from our poor health to our inflated sense of readiness. The real tragedy, however, is that this was so preventable. Not only has this pandemic long been expected, but the exact manner in which it played out was predicted as well. Yet, we still failed to believe it or act on the information we had available until it was too late. When the coronavirus task force did another tabletop exercise in the underbelly of the West Wing's Situation Room on February 21, 2020, as the pandemonium of the scourge was taking deep root, the conclusion was obvious as Dr. Fauci recalls from the crucible of this war: "We're in for a disaster."

CHAPTER 2
MULTISYSTEM ORGAN FAILURE

A month before the tabletop exercise that capped The Lost Month of February, Dr. Carter Mecher, a senior medical adviser at the Department of Veterans Affairs for the Office of Public Health, had typed an email to a small, elite group of public health experts warning them that the WHO and CDC "were behind the curve" in responding to the novel coronavirus and swift action was needed to stop it. The recipients, all of whom held high-ranking positions in the government or at universities, belonged to a group jokingly nicknamed Red Dawn, a nod to the 1984 movie that pitted actors Patrick Swayze and Charlie Sheen against a foreign enemy invasion. The "Red Dawn Breaking Bad" email thread was hosted by Dr. Duane Caneva, chief medical officer at the Department of Homeland Security.*

* The *New York Times* did a marvelous job report-

Caneva wrote that the chain was started "to provide thoughts, concerns, raise issues, share information across various colleagues responding to COVID19."[1]

Mecher's email that night on January 28 was stark: "This is really unbelievable. . . . Any way you cut it, this is going to be bad. . . . The projected size of the outbreak already seems hard to believe." Mecher had analyzed early data from China and concluded that the virus was as transmissible as the flu, but with a greater ability to replicate and a case fatality rate far worse. "You guys made fun of me, screaming to close the schools," Mecher wrote. "Now I'm screaming, 'Close the colleges and universities.' "

Dr. James Lawler, an infectious disease doctor at the University of Nebraska who served in the White House under President George W. Bush and as an adviser to Presi-

---

ing on the Red Dawn emails based in part on Freedom of Information Act requests to local government officials. It has published more than eighty pages of the exchanges, which started in January 2020 and provide a diary of sorts for experts reacting to the spread of the coronavirus. You can download the file at www.nytimes.com. Some of the emails were also reported by Kaiser Health News.

dent Barack Obama, was also a regular participant in the email chain. He too predicted the gravity of the situation and followed with his own not-so-subtle bomb on the Red Dawn chain a few hours after Mecher:

From: James V. Lawler
Sent: Tuesday, January 28, 2020 8:56 PM
Great Understatements in History:

Napoleon's retreat from Moscow — "just a little stroll gone bad"
Pompeii — "a bit of a dust storm"
Hiroshima — "a bad summer heat wave"

AND

Wuhan — "just a bad flu season"

This was the same day national security adviser Robert O'Brien warned President Trump that this would be "the roughest thing" he'd face.[2] Matthew Pottinger, the deputy national security adviser, agreed and shared his own dire warnings with the president after reaching personal contacts in China. Pottinger would know: He had worked as a journalist in Hong Kong first for Reuters and then the *Wall Street Journal* during the SARS epidemic, later becoming a Marine Corps intelligence officer. During his years in China, he'd collected a handful of trusted friends he could rely on at this pressing time. He was the White House's foremost China expert and was attuned to the Communist regime's dishonest behavior and lapses in biolab safety.

According to Pottinger, the Chinese government was not telling the truth and had handed over the crisis to its military — not their own CDC with which the US CDC worked.[3] Once the Chinese CDC was cut out of the emergency, the Chinese military went about trying to cover up and contain the crisis. It also meant that our CDC director, Bob Redfield, who had been in regular contact with his counterpart, Dr. George Gao, the Chinese virologist and immunologist who led China's version of the CDC, was also out of the loop. According to Redfield, the Chinese government was lying not only to the world, but to its own doctors and public health authorities.

DECEPTION OUT OF CHINA

When I sat down with Redfield in 2021 to get his perspective on the previous year, it was a snowy February day. He had recently left his post at the CDC and was back in

Baltimore sorting through boxes from the move and piecing his life together again as a private citizen. Redfield told me they'd put in several requests to be allowed into China, including President Trump appealing directly to President Xi Jinping. All were denied. One of Redfield's biggest regrets was not successfully gaining entry to China in those early days. He couldn't get his CDC people deployed from Beijing to Wuhan to start a formal investigation. Instead, all he could do was have regular discussions with his friend Gao. Their private conversations, likely recorded by the Chinese military, revolved around the truth about this new pneumonia and how it spread. For example, when Redfield noticed that the first twenty-seven individuals in China diagnosed with COVID were comprised of three distinct clusters, he knew that meant these people were infecting each other as opposed to all contracting it independently from another location or walking through the same market. This was a clear sign of human-to-human transmission. On a call in the first week of January, Redfield remembers pointing out the obvious: "George, you don't really believe that mother and father and daughter all got it from an animal at the same time, do ya?"

Inexplicably, George's reply was along the lines of: "Bob, there's just no evidence of human-to-human transmission."[4]

Redfield challenged his friend of twenty-odd years, describing cases that had nothing to do with the wet market. The Chinese government and military had long been controlling the narrative and keeping the focus on the wet market, unbeknownst to him. Gao did not even know that there had been an outbreak of respiratory illness in the Wuhan Institute of Virology (WIV) back in the fall of 2019 (the antibody testing of those lab workers did not reveal coronavirus exposure, but those lab results were not independently confirmed). Three researchers from the lab got sick enough to seek hospital care.[5] This was weeks before Beijing later said its first confirmed case was a man who fell ill on December 8.[6] Had Redfield been able to better assist his friend with twenty or thirty people on the ground in those first few weeks in January, he thinks the pandemic's plotline would have changed.

Gao finally realized the enormity of the situation one night on another private call with Redfield. Gao broke down, audibly and tearfully distraught after finding "a lot of cases" in the community who had never visited the wet market. He knew the situation was not only out of his control, but people were dying, and the crisis was being directed by the higher-ups in government and the military, and that likely had been going on awhile. The initial mortality rates in China were somewhere between "5 and 10 percent," Redfield told me. "I'd probably be cryin' too," he added. (To this day, we don't know how many Chinese citizens were infected or died; the numbers could be grossly undercounted.)

During my postmortem conversation with Redfield, it became apparent that he was very concerned about Gao's safety and was protective of him. At times, Redfield leaned forward conspiratorially and told me that he was worried about George Gao's security, and he wanted to say nothing that could incriminate him in the eyes of the Chinese government, which he doesn't trust. It was arresting to hear a chief scientist so distressed that his friend and Chinese counterpart might be physically harmed just for revealing the scientific evidence he was uncovering. When Gao and Redfield spoke in early January, it was clear that while China's CDC was far out of the loop, the country's central government knew what was going on and was secretly preparing for the spreading disaster: It was at least a month ahead of the rest of the world in terms of securing N95 masks and other PPE, reagents for testing, and the development of vaccines — the essentials they'd need to manage a pandemic. They were buying up these supplies before alerting the rest of the world.

There was other evidence the Chinese knew and were not telling. Toward the end of January, as we all watched the Chinese hastily build two massive coronavirus hospitals in just over a week, people like Redfield and Fauci thought, *Wait a minute. Why are you building hospitals overnight if you are not that worried?* Thousands of miles away, Debbie Birx was watching the international news in dismay one night over dinner in South Africa, where she was acting in her role as global AIDS coordinator for the President's Emergency Plan for AIDS Relief program (PEPFAR). The mere sight of sick people overwhelming hospitals and the need for new ones to be built rapidly was enough of a signal that broad-based community spread had been happening, and probably for some time. She and her colleagues found themselves yelling at the TV: *This is going to be a pandemic!*

Soon after, Redfield was handed a report

from his own CDC's internal modeling for the pandemic: The United States would have 2.2 million people dead by September. It made Redfield pause in shock, and later that night, his wife shuddered to think it meant one of them would probably be dead by the fall.

"JUST A BAD FLU SEASON"[7]

The one factor Crimson Contagion didn't account for was the nature of COVID. The covert experiment modeled the pandemic response after influenza — not a coronavirus like COVID that can have a long incubation period during which a person is infectious or, worse, asymptomatic throughout the active infection. That is precisely what set COVID apart from other pandemics and partly explains our chaotic, slipshod reaction to it. We were groping in the dark for weeks. And in that darkness, our missteps and oversights started to metastasize into one of the worst responses in the world. According to Redfield, "Early on the focus was symptomatic cases — case identification, isolation, and contact tracing. But it became very clear to us in late February that, unfortunately, the major mode of transmission of this virus was not symptomatic transmission. And that changed the whole ballgame."

We eventually learned that COVID was much deadlier than the flu and much more easily transmissible than either of its close cousins, SARS and MERS. We came to terms with the reality that aerosolized particles and asymptomatic carriers are significant drivers of its relentless spread. Everyone I spoke to who was part of the initial task force shared with me that their "oh no" moment was when it became suddenly clear and unmistakable that asymptomatic spread was happening with this virus. COVID created millions of modern-day Typhoid Marys, unwitting silent carriers of a deadly disease. Dr. Birx was especially unnerved by the realization this bug had secret superpowers that nobody acknowledged in its flight out of the gates. But she quickly saw the parallels to her decades-long experience in sub-Saharan Africa combating the AIDS epidemic.

Human immunodeficiency virus (HIV), the virus that causes AIDS, has surprising similarities to COVID even though they are very different. Both have an asymptomatic phase, although for HIV, it can be eight to ten years. With COVID the asymptomatic phase may be eight to ten days. So if you rely on people entering emergency rooms or coming to the hospital, you're already far behind in finding and stopping the community spread. Without proactive testing, by the time the first person develops severe illness, there is an avalanche of cases aggressively spreading the virus. Birx remembers the rapid spread of the infection on the cruise ships as particularly alarming: When nearly half of the passengers and crew end up positive for COVID and were asymptomatic when tested, that's a major clue the virus is an aggressive and stealthy predator.

That's exactly what happened on the *Diamond Princess* that docked for quarantine in Yokohama, Japan, on February 4, after a passenger fell ill and disembarked on January 25 in Hong Kong.[8] That passenger, an eighty-year-old man, is thought to have been the only carrier — patient zero — of the virus onboard, whose infection wound up spreading to 712 others, 14 of whom died. A staggering 50 percent of people aboard got the virus from a single source. When the CDC mapped out the spread of the infections onboard, they discovered that lines of cabins sharing plumbing created a vehicle for the virus's propagation: the toilets aerosolized the virus. People who had never shared physical space with infected passengers were nevertheless exposed.

Between March 1 and July 10, the CDC discovered nearly 3,000 cases of COVID or suspected COVID and 34 deaths across 123 ships.[9]

The virus's silent spread meant it was allowed to circulate a lot earlier before being detected. By many accounts, the virus started transmitting somewhere in early fall 2019, and local health officials in China had miscalculated their ability to contain it. This would be the second factor that worked against our pandemic response. First, the deliberate misinformation coming from China; and then came the cover-up.

Yale-trained epidemiologist Dr. John Brownstein, a professor of biomedical informatics at Harvard Medical School and chief innovation officer at Boston Children's Hospital, has some of the most captivating proof that the virus was sickening people as early as autumn 2019, months before the rest of the world was made aware. Canadian-born Brownstein, as ebullient and youthful as your favorite tenth-grade biology teacher, is a pioneer of digital epidemiology — leveraging diverse digital data sources to understand population health. He has advised the WHO, the Institute of Medicine, the US Departments of Health and Human Services and of Homeland

Security, and the White House on real-time public health surveillance data and has authored over one hundred articles in the area of disease surveillance.

Brownstein enlisted the power of both microsatellite technology and Internet search trends to "see" the first ripples of illness hit Wuhan before others took notice. Satellite images showed increasingly filled hospital parking lots in the late summer that didn't resemble the same lots in years past. There was also an uptick in searches of keywords associated with infectious disease on China's Baidu search engine (Baidu is Google's rival in China; because Google is essentially banned in China, Baidu is the chosen search engine). Satellite data like the ones Brownstein used have historically been employed not only by intelligence agencies but also the private sector. Day traders, for example, track traffic patterns in parking lots at places like Walmart and Home Depot so they can more easily get an idea of the goings-on and capitalize on their buys and sells. The data help inform their trades. These photographs can be taken every hour to show when volume in the stores is high versus low. Such technology has also been used to track respiratory diseases. Brownstein himself published a piece years ago that showed that hospitals in Latin America got superbusy during flu season. "You could predict flu season just by looking at the parking lots," he told me.

Using images from October 2018, Brownstein's group counted 171 cars in the parking lots at Tianyou Hospital, one of Wuhan's largest. Satellite data a year later showed 285 vehicles in the same lots, an increase of 67 percent. And there was as much as a 90 percent increase in traffic during the same time period at other Wuhan hospitals. In his paper, posted on Harvard's DASH server, his team writes, "Between September and October 2019, five of the six hospitals show their highest relative daily volume of the analyzed series, coinciding with elevated levels of Baidu search queries for the terms 'diarrhea' and 'cough.' "[10] While searches for "cough" typically increased at the beginning of yearly flu season, "diarrhea" was more closely linked to this pandemic. It's a twenty-first-century way of predicting the beginning and trajectory of an outbreak based on the behavior of large populations.

Not seeing those first cases to help us realize the nature of COVID cost us. Our learning curve grew steeper every day we didn't know, and we finally woke up to the reality after the nightmare began — which brings me to the third strike against us in our ability to manage the pandemic: testing failures. "Don't start preparing when you're in the middle of a pandemic," Dr. Brett Giroir said to me in my postmortem with him. Giroir, a pediatrician by training, is a former four-star admiral in the US Public Health Service Commissioned Corps and was the sixteenth assistant secretary for health from 2018 to 2021. He was named the testing czar early in the pandemic. "You can't create something out of nothing," he said. He mentioned a case in point: "We've been investing in vaccines for 20 years and we've reaped the benefit of that investment. But for testing, it wasn't ever mapped out or gamed beforehand so we couldn't achieve those goals on the fly. . . . We didn't have a resilient public, private, commercial, and academic infrastructure that could coordinate and work cohesively."

TESTING, TESTING, FAILURES 1-2-3
Testing too little, too late, was our original sin in the response. When COVID got stuck in a flu model early on, testing simultaneously suffered. "We don't really diagnose flu," Birx pointed out. "We treat flu by the symptoms during flu season. When you come down with a flu-like ailment during

flu season and you call your doctor, you'll likely be prescribed flu treatment without a flu test. With COVID the situation was not like flu — it was like HIV, with a large volume of asymptomatic people perpetuating the virus's replication and spread. And to deal with that, you needed to have testing."

Within the first ten days of knowing the virus's genetic sequence, the CDC sent out test kits it had developed. But they didn't work. Although the WHO had developed a test before the CDC, one that many countries were using, the United States chose not to use it and instead waited for its own testing system to become established. But that never really happened, at least not to the extent necessary to shove back against the virus's proliferation. As Birx put it to me, "We let the perfect be the enemy of the good." Instead of pushing to an impossible "perfect," and therefore getting nowhere, we should have accepted "good enough" and at least gotten somewhere. Many things worth doing are worth doing badly — even, and especially, in a pandemic.

Redfield was reticent to shoulder any of the blame for his agency's testing failure, even saying at one point that the CDC should have been congratulated on at least attempting to create the tests. The specifics to the flawed CDC tests are complicated and have been detailed in many news reports; suffice it to say they originally worked at the CDC but not in most public and academic labs where they produced inaccurate and inconclusive results. The CDC's recall of these tests caused a significant delay in testing — five weeks, The Lost Month, and then some. During that time, the virus was burning through our population as other countries were successfully deploying tests of their own. The mistake in these first-generation kits marred the entire testing enterprise from the start and put testing perpetually behind. Nobody wanted to talk about the misfire; even when I probed Redfield about it, he praised the CDC's record-time test development but grumbled at the harsh scolding his center received for testing failures on the ground. People unrealistically expected the CDC to test hundreds of millions of swabs every week and produce those hundreds of millions of test kits. But the center was not equipped for such a monumental task; it simply didn't have the manufacturing capacity to provide that number of kits, let alone perform the kind of testing we all knew was needed for mitigation — especially when it involved an epidemic bolstered by asymptomatic spread.

"We needed a Manhattan Project for testing," Redfield now notes in retrospect. He can identify the holes easily that were not about to be filled instantly when the pandemic hit, and surely not by a single organization or individual. These are holes that take decades to plug and then build on: A public health infrastructure at the ready for a pandemic, robust data analytics and reliable predictive data analysis, laboratory resilience, and a public health workforce in every health department in the country that's ready to respond to a deluge of cases. Although the CDC, which is based in Atlanta, Georgia, and has employees in more than sixty countries and forty American states, is tasked with protecting the country from infectious disease threats, it's surprisingly limited in its ability to order actions. It provides funding for most of our state, local, and tribal public health departments, as well as information and guidelines, but those do not translate to mandates. (An interesting aside: The CDC was founded in 1946 to prevent the spread of malaria across the country as veterans carried it home after World War II.)

Birx stressed the importance of rigorous

proactive testing in the first set of gating criteria — the benchmarks on the way to reopening after the nation paused in March. These benchmarks had to be data driven. Who is infected? Who is sick? Who needs treatment? You have to routinely test staff in nursing homes, county health workers, and so on in order to see the epidemic and your imminent surge *before* that first person is hospitalized. "And if you work in a hair salon," Birx told me, "you have to be regularly tested — not because we believe that you're a huge risk to the clientele, but because you are in the public." These individuals are like our sentinel surveillance people who act as beacons on where the virus is lurking and how we should respond. Unfortunately, the value of aggressive testing never sunk in at the White House.

Another huge misfire around tests occurred over the summer when the CDC issued guidance on its website telling people that they didn't need to be tested if they were asymptomatic. This was around the same time Trump and his advisers, including Dr. Scott Atlas, a radiologist by training who didn't believe in testing for asymptomatic cases, seemed to be pushing for a slowdown in testing. People in the White House believed that testing was driving cases rather than slowing them down. By slowing testing, they could make the COVID numbers look better — which is like wearing a turtleneck over a massive lump in your neck to avoid acknowledging what could be serious. At some point, you have to look squarely at the lump and deal with it. Or you're playing dumb. Redfield says he was never explicitly told to slow testing. Trump's comment at a Tulsa campaign rally, where he said to the audience he'd asked his people to "slow the testing down please" because "when you do more testing you find more cases," was later explained away as "semi–tongue in cheek." But all this muddled messaging would end up being unhelpful, and deadly. The CDC's guidance was revised within twenty-four hours due to its risk of being "misinterpreted," to use Redfield's word. Mixed messaging was yet another strike against us.

MIXED MESSAGING
IN A POLITICAL MIRE

For Redfield, the most egregious move by the White House in the pandemic response came when he says he was aggressively pressured to tamper with the CDC's most important and prestigious publication, the *Morbidity and Mortality Weekly Report*

(MMWR), a weekly epidemiological digest for the United States. Authored by career scientists and approved by the director, the MMWR is the main vehicle for publishing public health information and recommendations that the CDC has received from state health departments. It has been a fixture in our public health landscape for decades and is considered one of the most revered publications health care professionals use to make important decisions, some of them in life-or-death scenarios. When you're in a pandemic, such a scientific report is critical because it informs doctors, researchers, and the general public about how a pathogen like COVID is spreading and who is at risk.

Claiming that the MMWR's COVID reporting was aimed at hurting the president's bid for reelection, Redfield told me the HHS Secretary Alex Azar and his staff, perhaps under the direction of the White House, asked that the reports be modified and, in some instances, delayed their publication. This was an absurd, if not unethical, proposed intervention. "Now he may deny that, but it's true," Redfield told me in reference to Azar's coercion.[11] The CDC director was not going to surrender to pressure — not when his name was going on these scientific reports. The MMWR was "sacrosanct" on his watch. On a drive home one evening, after pushing back on the Office of the Secretary in a heated dialogue that lasted for at least an hour, the call came in again. This time, it was Alex Azar's lawyer and his chief of staff. They wanted certain details changed in the MMWR.

"We agreed that you're gonna do this," came the curt directive from the other end of the line, Redfield recalled. They squeezed Redfield's tolerance for psychic pain for another hour. They "dumped on him good," accusing him of being out of line and asking him to write a foreword in the MMWR that was different from the report's findings. Redfield told them that CDC directors don't write editorials in these science-backed, vetted reports — especially editorials that contradict and obfuscate the facts and data. There would be no change in editorial policy, Redfield countered to their demands. Most important for Redfield, however, this was his breaking point. After endless badgering, he drew the line and called out their professional harassment. If they wanted a director who would change the MMWR, they'd need to get another director. Redfield told me, "I finally had a moment in life where I said, 'You know, enough's enough. You wanna fire me?

Fire me.' And I just said, 'I have to let you all know I'm recording this conversation.' "

He wasn't recording the conversation other than implanting the memory in his own head. But pretending he was documenting the heated exchange was Redfield's reflexive way of pushing back without quitting. (In a statement, Azar denied putting any pressure on Redfield to revise the reports.)

I asked Redfield the question: Why didn't you quit? Even his children were suggesting he resign in the spring. One of his sons, a transplant surgeon, called a lot and nudged his father to quit, but Redfield refused. He reminded his son of the *Don't Quit* plaque, which his son had given him years ago. "God must've had a reason for you to give me this plaque," Redfield told his son, "so I'd be able to read it back to you at this moment in time." The unfortunate role that politics played in the American response has led Redfield to urge that leaders at places like the CDC, NIH, and FDA be appointed for seven to ten years so they are less politically aligned with a single presidency or party. He mentioned the example of the FBI, whose director is appointed for a single ten-year term by the president and confirmed by the Senate.

When Birx moved from the State Department over to the White House, leaving Africa and accepting her position as the coronavirus task force coordinator, she found herself among people "who did not take the pandemic seriously." And she knew taking the job was career suicide. Her first order of business, nonetheless, was to understand the culture so she could then try and make government work efficiently and effectively. But she arrived in the middle of the mess, like a bird touching down on a branch of a tree that has already been uprooted by the violently swirling storm. Her efforts in mid-March to push the administration to declare a fifteen-day time-out to slow the spread came only after many sleepless nights and data presentations with easy-to-read charts and graphs that would persuade Trump and his aides. And when it was abundantly clear at the end of March that another thirty days would be necessary to slow the spread, Birx endured another round of sleepless nights, consultations with Fauci, and grade school chart making to show and convince the president.

By then, people in Trump's circle were increasingly nervous about what the lockdown would do to the economy. In the end, though, it may not have been the detailed presentations that convinced the president to extend the pause. Trump likely agreed because he had friends dying from the infection, and that may have made this real for him personally. After that second pause, however, Birx was thought to have apparently overstayed her welcome in the eyes of Trump's coterie and was largely sidelined. She'd never brief the president directly again. "The one policy directive he gave to me in April, which was the last time I really had any briefing with him in that kind of way, was, 'We will never shut the country down again,' " Birx said.

In mid-May the administration sought to artificially attribute some deaths to other causes, skeptical of the CDC's reporting and hoping to keep the numbers down.[12] Debates about how to count the deaths ensued, particularly when it came to people dying with underlying conditions that alone could have been life-threatening. But even when a person lives with heart disease, for example, and then dies soon after contracting the virus, it's COVID that took that life. You can't cover up COVID deaths. Or, for one more example, if you go into the hospital for cancer treatment and come out in a coffin because you picked up an infection while there, your death certificate will list "septic shock" due to that infection first as the cause of death.

Over the summer, as Scott Atlas's extreme ideas about controlling the pandemic, which included letting the infection rip through younger people, ran counter to the rest of the task force, the chaos continued. Atlas questioned the effectiveness of masks too, which went directly against the task force's messaging. Birx noticed the president was receiving a parallel stream of data, likely from Atlas's team, that did not jibe with her own data. They were slicing and manipulating the data to try and show that the United States was doing better than Europe. The messages coming from the White House no longer reflected the science-backed truth. "We mitigated too late and opened too early," Birx said to me in our postmortem analysis. "We didn't communicate effectively. We need to be better marketers of our message. Our federal messaging was not consistent, and the way you talk to a twenty-something or middle-aged individual, someone in the heartland versus people in New York City or L.A., is very different. If you have 100 messages and 99 percent of them are on focus and 1 percent is off, it only takes that one message to lose trust and create doubt. And that really causes a problem."

Birx realized how bad the messaging was when she met with communities that had misinterpreted important information that influenced their behavior and adherence to public health measures. In some of the Rocky Mountain states, for example, the CDC found that 94 percent of people who died from COVID had underlying conditions (what are called *comorbidities*). The headlines at the end of August were everywhere: "CDC Says 94% of COVID-19 Deaths in US Had Underlying Medical Conditions."[13] That led to a claim that went viral within days on social media: that only 6 percent of US pandemic deaths had been from COVID itself. People took a mental shortcut that resulted in faulty causal thinking. They thought the headlines meant the vast majority of people who died from COVID actually died from causes other than COVID so that gave them permission, they decided, to avoid public health guidelines like mask wearing, or at least not take them seriously if they didn't have any underlying conditions. It wasn't that they were antiscience — they were misunderstanding the data and, in turn, what they were supposed to do. Mind you, a lot of people do have risky underlying conditions like high blood pressure and being overweight or obese but either don't know it or don't acknowledge it.

Such a fallacy of logic over these percentages and resulting risk assessments would be like concluding 90 percent of the people who died on 9/11 died of heart disease, diabetes, or stroke. Yes, there is a lot of chronic, preventable illness in the United States, and that is a problem we need to confront as a nation. But there were more than half a million excess deaths during the first year of this pandemic (522,368 excess deaths to be exact, according to the *Journal of the American Medical Association*).[14] Those are mothers, fathers, sons, and daughters who would have still been here — even with their conditions to manage — but are now gone. The misunderstanding led to people downplaying the virus in their heads and behaving counter to guidelines. They simply didn't understand the data that were informing the guidelines. The confusion only compounded our political divides. Rather than uniting to attack a common enemy — the virus — we seemed to fight with one another. But as you're about to find out, viruses don't pick a political party.

They don't even pick a fight. They just . . . are.

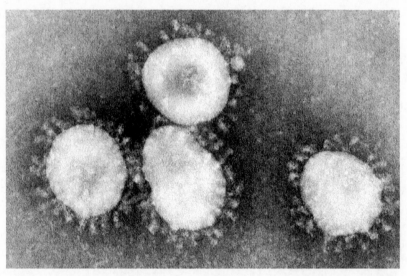

This 1975 transmission electron microscopic (TEM) image shows human coronavirus particles. Coronaviruses possess a helical genome composed of single-stranded RNA. The coronavirus derives its name from the fact that under electron microscopic examination, each virion is surrounded by a corona, or halo, due to the presence of viral spike structures emanating from its envelope. SOURCE: CENTERS FOR DISEASE CONTROL AND PREVENTION (DR. FRED MURPHY AND SYLVIA WHITFIELD).

CHAPTER 3
SNAKES

April 1, 2020

I wish the news had been different. But it was no joke. On April Fool's Day, as the pandemic was gaining strength and wizardry in our communities, I was mourning the loss of a dear colleague and friend while putting my thoughts together for a written tribute. Dr. James T. Goodrich was a giant of neurosurgery best known for performing the delicate and daunting operation of separating twins conjoined at the head.[1] These separations, which involve months of planning and dozens of procedures, are among the most challenging in medicine. I know, because I was with him for twenty-seven hours as he led a courageous team of forty doctors and nurses to operate on Jadon and Anias McDonald and allowed my crew to document the remarkable event, his seventh separation procedure of his long career. Even as a neurosurgeon myself, I had never seen anything like it.

Our shared world of neurosurgery is a small one. There are just 4,600 neurosurgeons in the United States, and as a result, we all cross paths at one point or another. I first met Dr. Goodrich when I was a resident, and even back then, he had a Santa Claus–like beard and a constant twinkle in his eye. He had a sly grin and always looked as if he knew the punch line of the joke before everyone else did. Along the way, we became close. He was a reader and could speak effortlessly about any topic I had on my mind. He was the kind of guy who performed these astonishingly complex operations on little babies' brains but also took time to bake cookies during the holidays and hand-deliver them to nurses. Given his stature as a preeminent pediatric brain surgeon, I loved watching people react when he told them he had dropped out of college at one point and became a surfer dude, as he described it. For many of us brain surgeons, he really was the most interesting man in the world.

That's why it knocked the wind out of me when I heard he had died early Monday morning on March 30. I knew it was only a matter of time before I'd learn of a death from COVID in my own circle, but I didn't expect it so soon, just a couple weeks after the pandemic had been declared. It felt particularly cruel and unfair. I knew this virus did not discriminate based on who you are or what you do, and yet I still could not believe it would rob the life of someone who had saved so many. I asked him once how he even first thought of performing craniopagus separations, and unsurprisingly, his answer was rooted in humility.

"If I had really done my homework and looked at the literature on craniopagus twins at the time, I would have never accepted them [as patients]. Because the literature was devastating," he told me. So, with a touch of cluelessness and lots of idealism, he plunged ahead into some of the riskiest and most technical operations one can perform on a human, let alone two humans simultaneously. All along, you might be forced to make the split-second, impossible decision to save one twin over the other. Dr. Goodrich spent more than thirty years at Montefiore Einstein in New York City where the "surfer dude" became the director of pediatric neurosurgery and a professor at Albert Einstein College of Medicine.

While I, like many others, had hoped to never know somebody who became ill or died from COVID that changed with Goodrich's death. A few days after his death, I learned of another one too close to home. Charlotte Figi, just thirteen years old, had inspired me to travel the world years ago in search of the truth about medical marijuana.[2] It led to my *Weed* documentary in 2013 that featured her remarkable transformation as she used medicinal cannabis to treat and manage crippling, catastrophic seizures. Charlotte was a little pioneer from Colorado whose legacy is having ignited the entire CBD movement today. To think she worked so hard to enjoy a full life and had much to look forward to, but then succumbed to an aggressive pneumonia that overtook her body. It was so early in the pandemic that COVID wasn't yet top of mind, and widespread testing wasn't available. Her mother, Paige, told me all the doctors were convinced it was the novel virus making its way across the country. I wept as I wrote a tribute for her as well.

By the time this pandemic is officially over, millions of stories like those of James and Charlotte — of people old and young — will be told and heard. Tears will flow and sadness will simmer. I thought about all of the lost souls on December 14, the first day someone in the United States was vaccinated. How could I not, for it was the day we could mark the beginning of the end. If only people like James and Charlotte, and countless others, had been able to steer clear of the virus and hold on long enough for its antidote.

V IS FOR VIRUS

The word *virus* has a funny origin. It denotes the venom of a snake and is derived from the Latin for "slimy liquid" or "poison."[3] It's a misnomer, really, because not all viruses are bad and result in destruction or death. In fact, viruses are necessary. Let me repeat that: Viruses are necessary, which I realize is hard to believe given how much this tiny strand of genetic material making up the coronavirus has traumatized our world. But viruses are the planet's dominant life-form. They have been an essential part of our very existence — and evolution — for millennia and have made significant contributions to our animal friends and those in the plant kingdom too. In cows, for example, it is a virus that changes the cellulose from grass into sugars that ultimately provide energy and facilitate the production of milk.

We've all been trying to avoid one particular virus in the pandemic, but as you read and breathe right now, viruses are entering your body unbeknownst to you — thousands by the day. They thrive in our oceans where, at last count, almost 200,000 different viral populations have been found from the surface down to more than 13,000 feet deep and from the North to the South Pole.[4] Think about that the next time you swallow a mouthful of seawater; you're gulping down about as many viruses as there are people in North America.[5] And many viruses flourish inside us, coating our gastrointestinal tract among other organs and tissues, where they serve important roles, such as destroying disease-causing bacteria. Bacteriophages, as they are known, are viruses that infect bacteria and act as soldiers on our mucosal surfaces such as the insides of the nose and mouth and the lining of the gut. You may have heard about the human microbiome — the sum of all microbes that live in and on us in a mostly symbiotic relationship. These commensal organisms, which include bacteria, viruses, and fungi, have contributed to our survival for millions of years and have evolved with us. The bacteria dominate, and their friendly role in our health, especially our metabolism and immunity, is at the forefront of medical research. The next frontier for medicine, in fact, will be unlocking the secrets to our library of viruses that also help us out — what's called our virome. Our virome is a lifelong companion. Collectively, our microbiome serves many functions that we haven't begun to crack yet scientifically (more on this in part 2).

World-renowned virus hunter Dr. Nathan Wolfe was among the Cassandras who years ago warned the world it wasn't ready for a pandemic and who could see COVID coming in his imagination. He has an obsession for what's called biological dark matter. According to him, we cannot even fully identify 20 percent of genetic material in our noses, and up to half of the genetic mass in our guts is "unidentified life."[6] I had always thought of that term *unidentified life* being used to describe alien life, not organisms inside my own body. Wolfe, whom you'll meet in part 2, is founder of Metabiota, a service to evaluate and manage biological threats for governments and corporations. In 2018, he had designed an ingenious insurance policy to help protect large businesses against massive financial losses due to a pandemic. Nobody bought it.[7]

We have four times more viral genetic material inside our genome than our own genes. And the part of our genome that codes for proteins ("genes") comprises only

2 percent of our DNA. We owe many ancient viruses for our ability to read, write, and remember. No, I'm not suggesting that viruses inside you right now are helping you to read this sentence as if they are butlers to your brain. But from a macrocosmic perspective, viruses that humans have encountered throughout evolution have become part of who we are at a molecular, genetic level, to the point where they've had a role in the development of our many cognitive skills and capabilities. They are, after all, pieces of information. They have shaped our DNA and acted as beneficial genetic parasites to give us better ways to think, form memories, and even build immunity. As previously noted, mammalian viruses can help protect against bad bacterial germs and act as anticancerous agents too. Other viral genes have been incorporated into our DNA on several different occasions throughout our evolution. The syncytin-1 gene from a retrovirus, for example (also known as *enverin*), encodes for a protein essential in the establishment of the placenta. In a way, we owe our ability to have children to ancient viruses.

We don't know how many species of viruses exist in the world, but it's suspected that the number is in the trillions. Of the few hundred thousand kinds of viruses that are known, fewer than 7,000 have names. Only about 250, including the new coronavirus, have the machinery to infect us. We aren't their only targets. Viruses infect mostly bacteria but also other animals and plants, from beans and blackberries to ticks and mosquitos, potatoes and bananas, birds, cats, and dogs. We have no idea where viruses came from originally, and scientists will forever debate whether they emerged before or after living cells on Earth.

The first known virus we ever documented scientifically was not one that infected humans. It decimated tobacco plants, turning their leaves a mottled dark green, yellow, and gray. In 1857, farmers in the Netherlands reported a disease sickening 80 percent of their crops. It spread so easily that touching an affected plant with a watering hose could damage the plant next to it. Martinus Beijerinck, a visionary microbiologist and botanist, had long thought the source was an infection of something entirely different from bacteria or a fungus. He called it *contagium vivum fluidum* (contagious living fluid), noting that the pathogen had the ability to slip through the finest-mesh filters that could trap bacteria, giving it almost liquid properties.[8] And this is how the word *virus* got unluckily attached to this peculiar class of germs. Beijerinck used the word *virus* from the Latin word for a liquid poison to label this new kind of pathogen. If it could pass through a filter normally used to capture bacteria, he knew he was handling something else — something much smaller. But he never deciphered the full virus story and never got a chance to glimpse them. Yet while he incorrectly thought viruses were liquid — they are technically particles — his results were nonetheless on target.

Beijerinck was known as a difficult, socially reclusive individual who refused to have his picture taken, verbally abused his students, and never dated or married; he believed that marriage would interfere with his work. But he was a scientific trailblazer with a keen ability for observation. He may not have earned points for his character, but he definitely earned his keep in the laboratory, conducting research until the very end when cancer took him at age seventy-nine. He is credited with being a prime mover in establishing general microbiology as a major field of study. Well before most universities recognized microbiology as a distinct discipline, he established the Delft School of Microbiology, which is now regarded as the ancestor for many such departments and institutions worldwide.

Plant pathologist Adolf Mayer, who was director of the Agricultural Experiment Station just east of Delft in the Netherlands' Wageningen municipality, began researching the tobacco blight in 1879 and named it the "mosaic disease of tobacco." Germ theory, the modern understanding that pathogens can make us sick, was slowly under development, but the concept of viruses would take time to be accepted and understood within a biological context. When Robert Koch, a German pathologist and one of the main founders of modern bacteriology, discovered the bacterial culprit behind tuberculosis in 1882, he developed a short guide for linking these bacteria to the diseases they cause. It would become known as Koch's postulates — the rules for recognizing the role of bacteria in illness: the bacteria had to be present in every case of the disease; it had to be isolated from the host with the disease and grown in pure culture; the specific disease had to develop when a susceptible host was exposed to a pure culture of the bacteria; and, finally, the bacteria had to be recoverable from that infected host.[9] (I should note that fewer than 1 percent of bacteria cause diseases in people.)

Mayer ran the experiments to see if this unidentified microbe met the criteria of Koch's postulates, but something wasn't right. Every time Mayer performed a cycle of germ isolations and reinfections to find the cause of mosaic disease, he failed. He could show that the sap from a sick tobacco leaf could pass the disease to a healthy leaf, but he couldn't produce a pure culture of the germ and couldn't spot the nemesis under a microscope. It was an invisible contagion.

Not being able to see viruses under an ordinary light microscope, like you can bacteria, made them elusive, confusing, unbelievable, and on the verge of fantastical. In 1929, American biologist Francis Holmes developed a method using the tobacco mosaic virus to prove that viruses are discrete particles and have stronger effects at higher concentrations. In essence, his method "made the virus visible" to some degree, but not like a photograph. It would take the invention of the electron microscope in 1931 to pave the way for imaging these exceptionally small microbes, which finally happened in 1935 by the American biochemist and virologist Wendell Meredith Stanley. He created a crystallized sample of the virus that could be "seen" with X-rays, earning him a share of the 1946 Nobel Prize in Chemistry.[10] The first unambiguous photographs of the tobacco mosaic virus would not be taken until 1941 with the invention of powerful transmission electron microscopes, which revealed the pathogen's skinny, rodlike shape. (Rosalind Franklin produced the clearest X-ray diffraction image of the tobacco mosaic virus in 1955, following her contributions to the discovery of DNA's double helix.)[11]

The visual proof was a turning point in science, dispelling doubts and quieting skeptics who had questioned the very existence of viruses. The images showed that viruses are simple structures made of genetic material wrapped in a solid coat of protein molecules (or, in the case of COVID, the virus is spherical and wrapped in a fatty envelope that makes them especially vulnerable to soap when you wash your hands). Although bacteria and viruses are both too small to be seen without a microscope, microbiologists will tell you that they are as different as giraffes are from goldfish. Bacteria are more complex, single-celled organisms with a tough exterior wall and a squishy beach ball full of fluid inside that cell. Most importantly, bacteria can reproduce on their own and have probably been around for 3.5 billion years. Viruses are tiny by comparison and can reproduce only by attaching themselves to a cell. Killing a virus isn't possible, because they aren't really alive. They are the zombies of the microbe world.

Whether we should call viruses "microbes" at all is up for debate. They cannot live on their own, contain not a single cell, and do not perform any kind of physiological task we usually equate with animal or plant life, such as eating, respiring, reproducing, and even dying. They are more akin to bits of data that need another piece of machinery — a host — to replicate and carry on. They are sacks of code sometimes called, ironically, capsid-encoding organisms, or CEOs. They don't grow or move; we help them get around. We are the giant computers that run their software programs in our system. And for COVID it's like a nefarious computer virus — a bad computer bug that takes over our controls and turns our system against us.

SON OF SARS
Human evolution has been slow and steady. It took the genome of the human species 8 million years to evolve by 1 percent. But

ask your fellow virus that wants to infect you how long it takes to make a few adaptive changes to its wardrobe, and it will say to wait a day. Viruses practically change with the weather. Many viruses that infect animals, including COVID, can evolve by more than 1 percent in a matter of days. Coronaviruses, which are single-stranded RNA molecules, accumulate mutations at a rate 1 million times faster than human DNA does. They are simple, small, and nimble, whereas we *Homo sapiens* are complex, large, and often clumsy.

For those who want to understand the difference between DNA and RNA, here's the briefest explanation. The two molecules are the power couple in all living organisms to sustain life and carry hereditary information, but they are not structurally identical. RNA is single stranded, like a ribbon, while DNA is double stranded and therefore more stable and sturdier. DNA looks like a twisted ladder, the one you memorized from your high school biology text. The chemical makeup or "ingredients" of DNA and RNA are also not identical. RNA nucleotides — the basic building blocks — contain ribose sugars, while DNA contains deoxyribose. And every scientist who studies this knows that uracil is specific to RNA, while thymine is present in DNA (don't panic: you will not be tested on this). The important point is that DNA and RNA are partners in serving the function of maintaining the blueprint of life, and their main job is to produce proteins, which are the key products in the support of life on Earth.[12]

In most organisms, DNA stores the genetic information for building living things and transmits those precious codes to offspring, while RNA is mainly involved in transferring the genetic code for protein synthesis — the body's manufacturing of proteins to support life. Proteins are the body's workhorses: They are required for the structure, function, and regulation of all tissues and organs. Put simply, proteins drive the chemical reactions needed to keep cells alive and healthy. DNA is mostly found in the nucleus of cells, whereas RNA is found in the surrounding cytoplasm. Until recently, RNA was thought of as merely a messenger between DNA and proteins, but RNA can do far more. Because RNA can drive chemical reactions, as proteins do, and carry genetic information, like DNA, most scientists think life as we know it began in an RNA world — without DNA and proteins. RNA and viruses likely coexisted for a long time before the more complicated

DNA molecule showed up in Earth's life story, or memoir.

Because the mutation rate for the RNA in viruses is exponentially higher than DNA, they have an extraordinary ability to survive an assault from our immune system — they can quickly undergo a wardrobe change or alter their spike proteins to be able to bind tightly to a human receptor to enter our cells, as in the case of COVID This is why we hear so much about variants — the mutant strains of COVID that have emerged and can render the virus more contagious or deadly. Viruses that spill over from an animal such as a bat to a human are called *zoonotic* viruses.

Today, three-quarters of all new infectious diseases affecting humans originate in animals, and at least thirty new infectious diseases have emerged in the past thirty years — including SARS, MERS, and now COVID. Collectively, they threaten the health of hundreds of millions of people. One of the more alarming reports by the United Nations states that on average, a new infectious disease appears in humans *every four months*.[13] There are many reasons for this, but the confluence of climate change, population growth, genetic adaptations in microbial agents, international trade and travel, and changes in land use is chief among them.

Outbreaks of rare infections like Ebola often make headline news, but more problematic are the highly communicable ones that spread via breathing, talking, whispering, kissing, hand-shaking, hugging, and singing. Given that they evolve so much more quickly than we do, our natural immunity is unlikely to keep up. And since we're increasingly encountering these viruses in nature, we have to get crafty at countering them with other strategies — vaccines being one powerful counterpunch, among others.

One feature of modern pandemics that makes them stand apart from those in previous centuries is that their origins are off the grid. For thousands of years, we owed the contraction of most of our infectious diseases to domesticated animals — livestock like pigs, birds, cows, and cattle. The common cold originated in camels, and many strains of flu come from pigs and birds, such as H1N1 and H5N1. Today, however, our pandemics spring from close encounters of the wild kind. Ebola has repeatedly jumped from bats to primates and humans in Central and West Africa. Middle East respiratory syndrome (MERS) leaped from bats to camels to humans in Saudi Arabia. In the United States, the CDC responded to an Ebola outbreak in imported macaques at a primate research center in Virginia in 1989 and to monkeypox in 2003 that spread in the Midwest from infected rodents imported from Ghana.[14] The sick rodents were housed near prairie dogs sold as pets at a facility in Illinois, and thereafter infected people. The new coronavirus's genome is 96 percent similar to a bat virus. How long ago it made the jump from a bat to a human, acquiring the mutations necessary to do so, is not known. The germ may have also hitched an intermediary ride through another animal such as a civet cat or pangolin before reaching human cells.

As a reporter, I have traveled to the epicenter of outbreaks in Southeast Asia and China, long known as hot spots for emerging infectious diseases. I saw how poverty, population density, changing agricultural practices, and proximity to wild animals can conspire to make outbreaks likely.

Proximity to birds has emerged as a major factor in the flare-up of diseases. Nowhere else on the planet do so many humans have such close contact with so many birds as in China. Ask any infectious disease expert where they'd predict the next outbreak's origin to be, and they will unanimously say China. At least two flu pandemics in the past century — in 1957 and 1968 — originated there and were triggered by avian viruses that evolved to become easily transmissible among humans. China is a hotbed for birthing modern pathogens. The comingling of multiple species cultivates ideal conditions for spreading disease through shared water, utensils, or airborne droplets of blood, saliva, feces, and other secretions. On Chinese farms, people and livestock often live close together, sharing their germs. Pigs can be infected by both bird flu and human flu viruses, becoming veritable mixing bowls for combining genetic ingredients and possibly forming new and deadly strains. The public's taste for freshly killed meat and the conditions at live markets, where stressed wildlife are stacked in wire cages and slaughtered on-site for buyers, create ample opportunity for humans to come in contact with these new mutations. You couldn't design a more perfect setting for the transmission of disease. It's the ultimate germ fest.

When COVID was first identified in late 2019, a video of a woman eating bat soup circulated widely on the Internet, sparking rumors that bat soup consumption in China caused the outbreak and the beginning of a barrage of misinformation. (As it turns out, the clip was taken in 2016 in the Republic of Palau, a country in the western Pacific Ocean, and the woman in the video was Mengyun Wang, a travel show host.) Still, there is no doubt that bats are prime reservoirs for new viruses, and there are a lot of them: A whopping one in four mammals on the planet is a bat, and 50 percent of mammals are rodents.[15] Hence, the source of most zoonotic infectious diseases are bats and rodents, with bats dominating. They carry more than sixty viruses that can infect us, including Ebola and rabies. They are the natural reservoir for the rare but grisly Marburg virus, and Nipah and Hendra viruses, which have caused human disease and outbreaks in Africa, Malaysia, Bangladesh, and Australia. Bats also carry more human pathogens than other animals. Why? Because like us, bats are highly social creatures that prefer to live close to one another, giving them plenty of opportunities to spread pathogens among them. They also often live in huge colonies in caves, where crowded conditions are ideal for passing viruses to one another. These caves are abundant in Southeast Asia and China.

What's more, the ability to fly makes their

power of infection wide ranging. It also may help them adapt to the viruses so they are unaffected by them. Indeed, the physiological requirements of flight amp up their immune systems, helping protect them from the viruses they harbor. Flight also causes bats to have heightened metabolisms that raise their core body temperature to about 38°C (or 100.4°F). This means that bats are often in a state that for humans would be considered a fever. Researchers have suggested this may be a mechanism which helps bats survive viral infections. As a result, these winged rodents often host these germs without suffering any health consequences. (You may be wondering why not just exterminate the bats, if they are reservoirs for so many terrible pathogens. It's not that easy. They are important players in our global ecology: they pollinate plants and rid the world of many pests. On top of that, they are excellent subjects for studies on healthy aging, cancer prevention, disease defense, biomimetic engineering, ecosystem functioning, and adaptive evolution.)

Because we humans haven't yet evolved an equivalent kind of biological technology to evade the effects of these potent viruses, human-preying germs like COVID are hugely damaging. When you die of an infection, it's often the result of your body's own inflammatory response — not the invading germ itself. It's friendly fire run amok. This has been the case for scores of people who succumbed to COVID. The germ foments a lethal blaze in the immune system — called a cytokine storm — that cannot be contained before it does lasting damage to organs and tissues. The ongoing cytokine storm may also play a role in those long-haul COVID patients who cannot shake the illness months after clearing the virus. It's like a hit-and-run accident. The virus invades the body, messes with its machinery and balanced functionality, and leaves it forever changed before it takes off in search of new hosts.

Coronaviruses are a family of viruses named because of their regal appearance with crown-like spikes on their spherical surfaces (*corona* is Latin for "crown"). Although this family of viruses didn't earn its name until 1968 when scientists finally isolated and glimpsed coronaviruses under the electron microscope for the first time, these infectious microbes have been around for millennia — possibly for hundreds of millions of years, predating us.[16] The first reported case of a coronavirus was in 1912, when German veterinarians debated the diagnosis of a feverish cat with an enormously swollen belly. They didn't know what was wrong with it, and further did not know that coronaviruses were also giving chickens bronchitis and pigs an intestinal disease that killed almost every piglet under two weeks old. The link between harmful pathogenic coronaviruses and these animals, humans included, remained a mystery until the late 1960s. Certain types of coronaviruses cause relatively benign common colds, while others mutate into more virulent forms, such as the coronavirus behind the quickly contained outbreak of severe acute respiratory syndrome (SARS) in the early 2000s. In fact, we didn't think coronaviruses could be so deadly to humans until SARS emerged, which had a case fatality rate of 11 percent, killing over half of people sixty-five and older who contracted it.

SARS is also a reason to take seriously the possibility that the strain of COVID that took the world by storm also came out of a lab, not a Chinese market. Here's why. In 2004, the SARS virus had been largely brought under control after only 8,098 reported cases worldwide and 774 known deaths.[17] The *Wall Street Journal* published a piece about a small resurgence of SARS tied to a safety accident.[18] Although the virus had natural origins, spilling over from bats to humans either directly or through animals like civets held in Chinese markets, some of the SARS infections were caused by escapees from research labs. SARS coronaviruses have a history of breaking out of laboratories in Singapore, Taiwan, and twice in Beijing. So what about COVID?

THE LAB LEAK THEORY

The "lab leak" theory is one that Jamie Metzl has long believed. He has been maintaining a thrilling diary of facts to make a strong case for the origins of COVID coming from the Wuhan Institute of Virology (WIV).[19] Metzl, with whom I worked in the White House during the Clinton administration, wears many hats and is a geopolitical expert on China. With a PhD from Oxford, a JD from Harvard Law School, and as a Phi Beta Kappa graduate of Brown University, his résumé is long and accomplished. He is also a wicked-fast triathlete, a man in a hurry. He has served at the US National Security Council, State Department, Senate Foreign Relations Committee, and as a human rights officer for the United Nations in Cambodia. In 2019, he was appointed to the WHO expert advisory committee on human genome editing. He is also senior fellow for technology and national security at the Atlantic Council, a think tank in the field of international affairs. He knows a thing or two about China and its hand in playing games with viruses. According to him, there's an 85 percent chance the pandemic started with an accidental leak from the Wuhan Institute of Virology and a 15 percent chance it began in some other way. He was one of the first in Washington, DC, to say the novel coronavirus could be a Wuhan lab escapee, and now he hopes to make the lab leak hypothesis an accepted possibility, not a conspiracy.

Wuhan is a city of 11 million people in central China, making it just the ninth most populated Chinese city. (Shanghai has 26 million people and Beijing 22 million.) Before COVID, you had probably never heard of Wuhan, but it has been on the science community's radar for some time because it is also home to the country's first BSL-4 lab (short for biosafety level 4). That is the highest biosafety level, reserved for labs that study the most frightening organisms — ones that are easily transmitted and highly fatal. BSL-4 labs are, for example, where extraterrestrial material would be studied. Laboratory workers don positive pressure suits, and everything they wear and touch is decontaminated (just as you see in the movies). Individuals go through chemical showers when exiting these labs, and if you look around, you won't find a single sharp edge that could cause an accidental tear in a glove or a gown. It's the kind of place where you would study organisms that have pandemic potential, such as bat coronaviruses, which is what this particular institute is known for doing. That said, it's been publicly acknowledged by the lab that prior to the pandemic, a lot of coronavirus research, including some involving live SARS-like viruses, had been conducted in less secure BSL-3 and even BSL-2 laboratories.

To be clear, Metzl is not suggesting the virus was totally genetically engineered or altered deliberately by mad scientists seeking to create bio-weapons. Nor is he dismissing the possibility it was purely born from nature outside the lab in a random leap from a wild animal to a human. But for him, the lab theory must be thoroughly investigated. He believes the bio-weapon that is COVID19 was born in nature but then possibly bred by science. It received an education to better infect humans. Dr. Bob Redfield, the former head of the CDC under Trump, believes this too. "It's not unusual for respiratory pathogens that are being worked on in a laboratory to infect the laboratory worker," Redfield told me. "And can you imagine if that laboratory worker then was asymptomatic? They wouldn't even know they were infected, right?" The implication is that a single asymptomatic person could be the tip of a pandemic-sized iceberg.

Redfield finds it implausible, if not impossible, that a virus could jump directly from an animal like a bat or civet cat to a human "and immediately become one of the most infectious, transmissible pathogens known to humanity." He explained to me that it doesn't make biological sense for a pathogen to go from a wild animal to a human and spontaneously be extraordinarily efficient at human-to-human transmission. It takes a while for pathogens to gain that level of fitness, or function. They sputter along for a while as they gain their athleticism to flex their muscles in human hosts. Like Metzl, Redfield finds it more plausible that the virus was being studied and educated in the lab, interacting with human cells — the training grounds for superb adaptation — before being accidentally unleashed on the public. "Most of us in a lab," Redfield explained, "when trying to grow a virus, we try to help make it grow better, and better, and better, and better, and better, and better so we can do experiments and figure out about it." It is often referred to as gain-of-function research — you tweak microorganisms in a lab in either petri dishes or other animals to make them more infectious. You teach it to do certain things. It's performed with the expectation that the transmission, and possibly the virulence, of the pathogen will be enhanced. Why would you do that? To stay one step ahead of the virus — to one-up mother nature. In nature, viruses don't want to become too lethal because if they kill their host, they "die" too. They reach a dead end, failing to multiply. Viruses devolve to something weaker, thereby surviving and proliferating. So when a bad virus gains a unique advantage to efficiently infect more and more humans, you have to wonder how it earned its wings.

"That's the way I put it together," Redfield concluded. He was clear that he's merely giving his opinion now that he's allowed to as a private citizen, but an opinion from the former CDC chief, who had access to raw data and intelligence gathering, is not the opinion of just any private citizen. Even Chinese scientists in Wuhan were raising concerns as early as January 2020, as two from separate universities asked an excellent question: How did a novel bat coronavirus get to a major city in the dead of winter when most bats were hibernating, and turn a market where bats weren't sold into the epicenter of an outbreak? Their resulting paper, which pointed to two local laboratories where research on bat coronaviruses took place, lived on the Internet for a blip in time before vanishing. We may never know how many papers like that as well as scientists and journalists were disappeared from China.

In January 2021, the WHO led a team of international scientists to Wuhan in search of the pandemic's origin. But after a full year had passed, much evidence was no longer available and the wet market in question had long been cleaned up and sealed off. It was a highly curated, chaperoned field trip hosted and controlled by the Chinese government, and its conclusions only led to more questions. Did the virus escape from the Wuhan lab where they'd been playing with coronaviruses for a while, and even working on their attachment to the same receptors in human cells as the COVID virus targets? We know this from published papers and research notes.[20] The institute has become a world leader on bat coronaviruses and has established one of the largest strain collections, but this lab also has a history of lax safety standards. The world's outbreak began right in its backyard. Its lab director, Dr. Shi Zhengli, published studies about manipulating bat coronaviruses in a way that could make them more infectious to humans.[21] Also known as "Batwoman" for her long history of hunting for coronaviruses in bat caves to study, Zhengli and her colleague Jie Cui are the ones who discovered that the SARS coronavirus likely originated in a population of cave-dwelling horseshoe bats in the Yunnan province in southern China. In their 2017 paper that reported their findings, they warned that "another deadly outbreak of SARS could emerge at any time."[22]

In another twist of prophetic irony, Zhengli had published a paper back in 2010 describing a scenario in which infected rodents led to a deadly virus being leaked from a Chinese lab. The paper, titled "Hantavirus Outbreak Associated with Laboratory Rats in Yunnan, China," reported on an incident in which an outbreak of the deadly hantavirus, which causes fever and kidney failure, occurred at a college in Kunming as the result of a lab leak in 2003.[23] In published interviews with Zhengli, she recalls thinking that when a coronavirus was identified as the cause of the pandemic, she wondered herself if it came from her lab.[24] To be clear, Zhengli's goals in studying these viruses and playing with their functionality do not necessarily have malicious intent. It's how scientists learn more about the virus's biological mechanisms behind its transmission and replication. It's also how we can discover possible mutations that may take place and ultimately allow better community surveillance, identifying when such mutations arise and permitting vaccines to be prepared in advance of such an outbreak. But clearly there's a fine line here that can cloud over.

Metzl has been critical of the 2021 probe, which allowed China to collect its own data and then hand it over to the WHO team, comparing it to tapping the Soviet Union to "do a co-investigation of Chernobyl."[25] He also enjoys quoting Humphrey Bogart from Casablanca: "Of all the gin joints in all the towns in all the world . . . why Wuhan?" Metzl highlights three facts that barely made the news. Number one: In 2012, six miners working in a bat-infested copper mine in Yunnan province were infected with a bat coronavirus. All of them developed symptoms exactly like COVID Three of them died. Number two: Viral samples from these miners were taken to the Wuhan Institute, the only level 4 biosecurity lab in China that was also studying bat coronaviruses. And number three: When COVID made its bona fide Wuhan appearance in late 2019, its closest known relative was the same virus sampled from the Yunnan mine where the miners had been infected.

The SARS outbreak nearly twenty years ago should have served as a wake-up call, showing us that coronaviruses can cause fatal respiratory illness and should not be ignored. It also exposed the real possibility of lab leaks. But it didn't prove to be a good enough villain: It didn't scare Americans because no one here died from it; only eight people in the United States were determined to have contracted the virus from traveling. It also didn't transmit easily during its relatively short, two- to seven-day incubation period. So even though scientists comparing the two viruses in recent studies determined that SARS was more lethal than COVID, it was not as contagious. COVID shares 79 percent genome sequence identity with SARS, but it is unique — and wicked — in its ability to infect. Indeed, the son of SARS has proven to be a far more social microbe, and it likes to travel quickly. It also takes its time to trigger symptoms in infected people who go on to develop the disease and show signs of illness. Meanwhile, these people are unknowingly infecting others — perpetuating the chain of transmission.

BIG AND STICKY

The RNA virus that causes COVID has a relatively large genome. Comprising a string of roughly 30,000 biochemical building blocks (again, these are called nucleotides) enclosed in a membrane of both protein and fat, it's more than three times as big as HIV and hepatitis C and twice the size of the average flu virus. But it's still tiny, coming in at barely one-thousandth the width of a human hair. This may be difficult to picture, but as Alan Burdick described it for the *New York Times*, "If a person were the size of Earth, the virus would be the size of a person."[26]

COVID is a savvy RNA virus. Its core code contains genes for as many as twenty-nine proteins, four of which give the virus its structure. The "S" protein, for instance, is of particular importance because it creates the spikes on the surface of the virus and unlocks the door to the target cell. This protein latches onto, or binds, to a receptor called angiotensin converting enzyme 2 (ACE2) on cells to gain entry. The S protein acts like a key inserting itself into a lock. The spike protein on COVID is nearly identical in structure to the one on SARS, but some data suggest that it binds to the target docking station far more snugly. It's sticky. Some researchers think this may partly explain why the new virus is so efficient at infecting us.[27] The other proteins encoded by the RNA serve various roles once the virus has entered a cell through the ACE2 cellular doorway. They hijack the cell's machinery and effectively turn off the cell's alarm system, commandeer the copier to make new viral proteins, and help the buds of new viruses shape and prime themselves for bursting out by the thousands to go on the prowl and infect other cells. If mistakes are made during the copying process and mutations occur, voilà — there's the birth of a new variant. Maybe it's more lethal or less, but rarely do variants lose their ability to perform their main function: infect, replicate, and spread. And repeat, over and over again. Often the variants that can infect more efficiently, as has been the case for the B.1.1.7. (Alpha) strain from the United Kingdom, become dominant strains; they can "run faster" to new hosts and outrun older strains, pushing them out of business. The Delta strain originally from India has also proven to be crazy fast and infectious.

Mutant strains of COVID will likely keep us hunting down the virus and firing at it with our vaccines, even though coronaviruses change more slowly than most other RNA viruses. That's probably because of a "proofreading" enzyme that corrects potentially fatal copying mistakes. A typical COVID virus accumulates only two single-letter mutations per month in its genome — a rate of change about half that of influenza and one-quarter that of HIV. Dr. Birx knows this territory well from her experience in the HIV world where variants foil attempts to control the HIV pandemic. "The virus is not thinking," she explained. It's not saying, *Hey, I should be better at getting into cells, so let's change the type of key I have so I fit better into the lock.* The virus is not proactively developing strategies and tools to infect us better or to escape our immune system and retaliatory attempts with drugs and vaccines. It's simply morphing under nature's forces, including the pressures we place on it. It has no plan or endgame other than to multiply. I love how Burdick sums up the real meaning of

COVID: "To know [COVID] is to know ourselves in reflection. It is mechanical, unreflecting, consistently on-message — the purest near-living expression of data management to be found on Earth. It is, and does, and is more. There is no 'I' in a virus."[28]

When you put immune pressure on a virus, whether through treatment or an immune response, induced by either monoclonal antibody infusions or vaccination, the virus randomly mutates. And if it finds a mutation that helps it multiply better, then that virus becomes the predominant virus. Birx has seen this with HIV in communities of spread, watching HIV change its wardrobe.

This phenomenon is the basis for molecular epidemiology, a study aimed at understanding and mapping the mutations in the virus's genetic sequence that give rise to the variants gaining dominance. I should point out that one of the key differences between HIV and COVID is that HIV never clears the body; it hides from the immune system, concealing itself in lymphocytes, or white blood cells, that are intrinsically hard to kill because they are resistant to killer T cells. Hence, HIV-positive patients remain positive because they are never cured. It remains a mystery why the body does not make an adequate immune response to HIV. COVID however, apparently persists until the body's immune system can deactivate the virus and clear it away, rendering a person negative if he or she can survive the effects of the infection.

Unlike the first SARS (sometimes called SARS Classic), which quickly finds a nice home in our lung cells with symptoms soon to follow, the son of SARS prefers to colonize quietly in the nose and throat before moving into the lungs. During this first phase of infection in the first week or so, a person may have mild cold-like symptoms (called paucisymptomatic) or no symptoms at (called asymptomatic) but still be highly infectious, shedding copious amounts of virus. The individual may develop a fever, dry cough, sore throat, loss of smell and taste, or head and body aches. Once the virus reaches the lungs, it's a whole new landscape as the infection enters a second phase. The delicate alveoli there — tiny sacs lined by a single layer of cells rich in ACE2 receptors — become compromised. The alveoli are responsible for trafficking the exchange of oxygen and carbon dioxide, so any compromise to them is a compromise to the whole body. The cascade of events that turns the lungs into a swampy mess can lead to pneumonia. For some, the infection steals so much of their breathing capabilities that they experience acute respiratory distress and need oxygen, sometimes a ventilator. Autopsies on COVID victims put on ventilators have shown that their alveoli became stuffed with fluid, white blood cells, mucus, and the detritus of destroyed lung cells.

The damage that COVID inflicts doesn't end with the lungs or respiratory system. In fact, no system in the body seems to be spared from potential insult, leading many scientists studying COVID's far-reaching effects to characterize it as a vascular disease. And those ACE2 cellular doorways are scattered prominently throughout the body in many cell types and tissues, including the lungs, heart, blood vessels, kidneys, bladder, brain, eye, pancreas, liver, and gastrointestinal tract. Because they are present in epithelial cells, which line certain tissues and create protective barriers, there is probably no organ or system in the body free of this critical receptor. It's even found in the prostate and testes, as well as the placenta. The ACE2 system is crucial to many biological processes, notably things like blood pressure regulation, wound healing, and inflammation. When the virus binds to and essentially clutters those ACE2 receptors, it prevents ACE2 from performing even the most basic critical functions.

The ubiquity of the ACE2 receptors partly explains how COVID can be so insidious far beyond the lungs and result in a perplexing array of conditions from head to toe. In addition to making the lungs ground zero (and a functional launch pad for spewing more viral particles to infect others), it can attack the lining of blood vessels and generate clots; harm the muscular walls of the heart; generate strokes, seizures, and inflammation of the brain; and hurt the kidneys. And one of the virus's greatest strengths appears to be its after-effects — the debris it leaves after the immune system has neutralized the virus. The actual virus may be gone, but it's not forgotten as the body remains stuck in a pro-inflammatory state. Future research will figure out why one person who contracts the virus experiences no symptoms while someone else is dead within days. Or why someone with a mild case goes on to have a long bout with a multifaced, prismatic illness. Or, most mysterious, how young children can develop chronic symptoms of illness months after an infection they never knew they had. The answers are probably not monochromatic. A complex constellation of factors — from purely genetic to environmental and the presence of preexisting conditions — is likely at play when it comes to explaining the vast spectrum of illness we've seen across individuals stricken with COVID. In fact, some studies are underway to determine if genetic differences in people result in how their ACE2 receptors function, putting one more or less at risk for a bad outcome from a COVID infection.[29] Variations of the ACE2 receptor could be a function of age, gender, and even ethnicity.

A question we now have to consider is this: Can COVID hide out in the body and continue to inflict damage? Can it persist long after the acute phase of illness has resolved? And could this be the cause of chronic symptoms in a subset of COVID long-haulers? Unfortunately, documenting persistent COVID infection isn't as easy as a repeat throat swab PCR or a simple blood test. Polymerase chain reaction, or PCR, is the laboratory technique used to amplify and detect genetic material from a specific organism, such as a virus. The PCR test to detect an active COVID infection in an individual is the "gold standard" for diagnosing the disease because it's the most accurate and reliable test, but you have to collect enough specimen for the test to work. It often takes invasive and painstaking measures to confirm a virus's ongoing presence, especially if it's hiding out in unsuspecting cells and tissues after the acute phase of infection. Such detective work is usually not available to patients outside a research setting. In many cases, we don't have proof that the virus is persistent — but we also don't have proof that it's not. Absence of evidence is not evidence of absence.

Studies are underway to understand how some viruses, including coronaviruses, could become persistent infections, and in some cases long after presumed recovery from the acute phase. The hypothesis that coronaviruses could linger in the body was suggested as far back as 1979.[30] And it remains to be fully documented how and where COVID can hide in places far from the respiratory system.[31] This highlights an important possibility: If the virus can remain in some people and cause chronic illness, then it similarly may not be gone in those who've experienced chronic illness after acute COVID, or the active phase of infection.

One case in particular that garnered attention in scientific circles and became a case report published in the *New England Journal of Medicine* involved a forty-five-year-old man with a severe, rare autoimmune disorder.[32] His condition had him on multiple drugs that suppressed his immune system when he contracted COVID in spring 2020. After a five-day stay at Brigham and Women's Hospital in Boston, he was discharged and quarantined alone at home for the next several months during which he was readmitted to the hospital multiple times for a recurrence of his infection. He was treated with many courses of antiviral medications and once with an experimental antibody drug.

Every time he thought he was free of the virus, he wound up back in the hospital, and he ultimately died from COVID after a grueling 154 days. The report that features the case calls attention to the obvious concern about people who harbor high levels of virus for months. The authors write: "Although most immunocompromised persons effectively clear [COVID] infection, this case highlights the potential for persistent infection and accelerated viral evolution associated with an immunocompromised state."[33]

One thing is for sure: If a pathogen wanted

to infect as many humans as possible, its doorman would be the ACE2 receptor, the COVID co-conspirator. This Bonnie and Clyde duo is perfectly paired to spread to as many people as possible across the planet and ravage as many bodies as possible. "The virus acts like no pathogen humanity has ever seen," wrote one group of scientists for the journal *Science*. [34] "Its ferocity is breathtaking and humbling." [35]

Tony Fauci described COVID's near-perfect adaptation to humans to me as if speaking from the virus's wise perspective:

Not only am I going to infect you, but I'm going to make sure that many of you don't have symptoms. And I'm going to make sure that those of you who don't have symptoms are going to account for 50 percent of the transmissibility. The people who are young and who are healthy, who don't get symptoms. I'm going to use them to spread as much as I possibly can because they're going to be well — they're not going to get sick and they're going to be infecting all their friends in this superspreader event. But I'm going to look for the vulnerables and the vulnerables are the elderly and those with underlying conditions. And if I kill the vulnerable, I'm not going to eliminate the population, so I always have a lot of people that I can still infect. . . . Now, that sounds crazy, but that's the metaphor that when you deal with infectious diseases, you say, *Damn!* This virus, it's such a bad evil virus because it's doing things in such a nefarious way. It's using transmissibility among otherwise healthy people and vulnerability of people who are going to wind up dying. It's a bad, bad virus.

On top of all that, people who cannot clear the virus can become breeding grounds for mutant strains, including individuals who never knew they were infected to begin with. Although the scientists studying the immunocompromised man with severe illness first wondered if he was merely acquiring new strains of the virus and becoming reinfected, they eventually determined that the same strain had been evolving over time in his body, acquiring a cluster of new mutations at an alarming speed. The man did make some antibodies in a feeble immune response, but his level of resistance was too low to clear the virus and just enough to put pressure on it. The virus was allowed to live in an environment where it had to change in order to survive.

Such scenarios are unusual, but they raise important questions we must address if we are to gain control of the variants and get ahead of the virus's attempt to thrive — which brings us to the topic of vaccines and their curative powers to prevent disease and end pandemics.

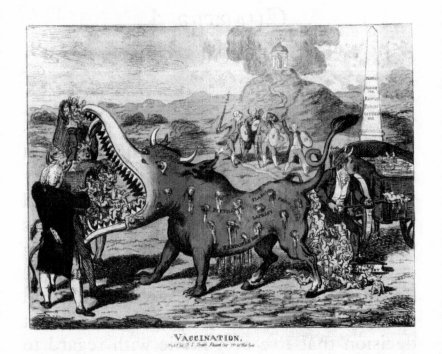

VACCINATION.

In this 1802 political cartoon, an etching by Charles Williams (1797–1830), vaccination was depicted as a diseased cow-like horned monster being fed baskets of infants and excreting them to symbolize vaccination and its effects. SOURCE: THE WELLCOME COLLECTION, LONDON.

Chapter 4
Cows

Three hours after the virus's code was published in January 2020, scientists around the world went to work to develop diagnostic tests and vaccines. Not a single case had been confirmed yet in the United States when Fauci ordered his team to get going on a vaccine. "The decision that we made on January the 10th to go all out and develop a vaccine may have been the best decision that I've ever made with regard to an intervention as the director of the institute," Fauci told me. It was a gamble, because an all-hands-on-deck approach to the vaccine development was going to be costly and there was no way of knowing at the time what would transpire. A "pandemic" had yet to be declared.

Although the skies looked clear, potential scenarios were playing in the back of Fauci's mind. The possibility that this would go bad, even though it wasn't going bad yet, was too hard to ignore. Fauci remembers the moment he trained his institute's efforts on a COVID vaccine. "I just turned to our people and said, 'Let me worry about the money. Just go and do it.' And boy, was that the right decision." By January 15, Fauci and his team were collaborating with Moderna on vaccine development. Sixty-three days later, they went into the phase 1 trial. "Just as we were going into the phase one trial," Fauci recalled, "count sixty days from January 10th, bingo, you're in the explosion in New York."

On a cold Sunday night in November 2020, Fauci sat bundled up on his deck, having a (physically distanced) drink with a friend when the call came. Albert Bourla, the CEO of Pfizer, was on the other end of the line. Pfizer had commenced its clinical trials in early May on a vaccine in development with BioNTech that, like Moderna, was based on the same technology. "Tony," Bourla said, "are you sitting down?"

Bourla had the results from the phase 3 trials that had been taking place for months after the first two phases. Bourla told him it was "amazing." I have known Dr. Fauci for twenty years, and he has always loved doing impersonations, and now he laughed as he mimicked Bourla giving him the news in a lyrical Greek accent. "Tony, it's more than 90 percent effective at reducing the risk of developing severe COVID!" Keep in mind that the FDA had set expectations earlier saying they would consider 50 percent efficacy worthy of authorization. In any given year, the seasonal flu shot is 40 to 60 percent effective. For a scientist like Fauci, it was a deeply emotional, cathartic moment.

A week later, Moderna divulged similar results.[1] Perhaps the most stunning thing about these two vaccines, which both rely on new mRNA technology, is how well they were shown to work across all age, racial, and ethnic groups. It's like having PPE, personal protective equipment, at a cellular level; it turns the human body into an internal vaccine factory.

If you were to ask a molecular biologist about these new mRNA-based vaccines, she would tell you that Cinderella has gone to the ball.[2] Always a beautiful technology, mRNA had largely been passed over until this moment, when it finally got a chance to shine brightly. Ever since we figured out the code of life, DNA, more than half a century ago, we've decoded a lot about the human body and the way DNA programs how we function and carry out our biological business. But research into DNA has not yielded actual defenses against disease. It is RNA research that has produced those. Not only are RNA-based vaccines being considered for all sorts of other diseases now, some of which have yielded to no other approach, but other pharmaceutical uses of RNA technology are now coming into their own as well, as I will describe later. And while you may fret and worry at the fact that these new vaccines are just that — "new" — they are born from decades of study. They take vaccine technology from an analog to a digital space.

In molecular biology, the discovery of DNA's double helix led to a universal truth: We owe our life to the relationship between how genetic sequences come together to code for proteins. And those proteins' characteristic shape stems from how various amino acids link together and fold. It's like language: Letters form words, which then form sentences whose meaning depends on how those words come together in a unique sequence and ultimately tell a story. The transfer of information from the cell's genomic library to its active physical inter-pretation (i.e., protein) depends on a partic-ular form of RNA that acts as a translator of sorts. The gene sequence is first copied from DNA to RNA; that RNA "transcript," or record of instructions from the DNA, is then edited to form a molecule called a messenger RNA (mRNA), which then goes on to make proteins — the ultimate product that supports and proliferates life.

In the twenty-first century, with horrendous diseases like smallpox and polio long gone or disappearing, people may fail to appreciate the power of vaccines. But vaccines may have done more good for humanity than any other medical advance in history. And because billions of people take them, they are also the most studied. "Vaccination is the most powerful gift of science from modern medicine," Dr. Bob Redfield emphasizes whenever he speaks publicly. And as Dr. Paul Offit, co-inventor of the rotavirus vaccine, shared with me, "We have largely eliminated the memory of many diseases." And without that memory, we easily underestimate or dismiss risks — until and unless we encounter them firsthand. The disappearance of vivid personal memories of polio, whooping cough, diphtheria, mumps, and measles has likely contributed to the rise of anti-vaccination sentiment in spite of the well-documented danger of these diseases.

Smallpox was among the most fearsome

diseases we have ever encountered and dates back tens of thousands of years, when it would routinely decimate large populations throughout Africa, China, and Europe. It may have been responsible for the death of the Egyptian pharaoh Ramses V, whose mummified head reveals classic smallpox scars. Later, smallpox scourged Western Europe, wiping out more people than the Black Plague, and landed in the United States along with European settlers. A century or so prior to a hint of the concept of vaccination, doctors in the seventeenth century found that scratching a bit of fresh material, or pus, from a smallpox pustule to an uninfected person under their skin, via a sharp lancet, would provide some protection against the illness. This was termed *inoculation,* from the Latin *inoculare,* meaning "graft."

When the English aristocrat and poet Lady Mary Wortley Montagu contracted smallpox in the early 1700s, she survived but was left severely disfigured. Her brother died from the disease. After she ordered that her children be inoculated, people who heard about the noble family's use of the technique started to think more positively about the concept of inoculation, though it would not be scientifically validated for about another half a century.

As is the case with many other ground-breaking discoveries, the smallpox vaccine, the first and most powerful of all, happened from a serendipitous and monumental observation. In the late 1700s, a small-town country doctor, Edward Jenner, noticed that farmers and milkmaids exposed to cowpox never seemed to suffer from smallpox during its frequent outbreaks. The milkmaids would retain their beautiful, blemish-free complexions after a brief bout with the illness, unlike those who either died from smallpox or suffered mightily and had a pockmarked face to show for it. Jenner began investigating if these workers were getting naturally vaccinated (*vacca* means "cow" in Latin) by exposure to the cowpox virus, which somehow provided protection against the smallpox virus.

Poxviruses are known to infect many animals, and cowpox was a common disease among cattle at the time of Jenner's observations, but produced much milder symptoms than smallpox, its more deadly relative. In 1796, Sarah Nelms, a young dairymaid, went to Jenner with cowpox lesions on her hands. After noticing the pustules were on the part of Sarah's hands she used to milk cows, Jenner inquired about the health of the animals. In fact, Sarah told him, a cow named Blossom had recently been infected with cowpox. Back then, there was no requirement to get approval from an independent review board to experiment and test his theory. So Jenner obtained some of the material from Sarah's pockmarked hand and scratched it into the arm of an eight-year-old boy, named James Phipps, the son of his gardener.

About a week later, Phipps developed temporary symptoms that included chills, a fever, some generalized discomfort, and loss of appetite. Two months later, Jenner conducted a risky human challenge trial, when he purposely exposed the young child to smallpox material. Keep in mind, this was a known deadly infection at the time, and no one was certain this would work or that the boy wouldn't succumb to the illness. I can only imagine the wave of relief when the boy stayed well, and Jenner concluded that his subject was protected from the deadly smallpox. Still, his idea of vaccination, scratching a small amount of cowpox virus into healthy individuals, was not an easy sell initially. But eventually people accepted the pricks in the arm — a vaccine that was itself a living virus named vaccinia and was delivered via a bifurcated needle. Most people born before 1972 have the telltale roundish, semi-sunken scar on their upper arm to show for it.

Unlike more modern vaccines, the smallpox pricks carried such a high viral load, injected just below the skin's surface, that a local infection of smallpox would occur, followed by the scar that could be up to an inch in diameter. After decades of worldwide vaccination, smallpox was declared eradicated in the United States in 1972, just a few years after I was born; in 1977 a single case of smallpox occurred in Somalia for the last time, and in 1980, the WHO considered smallpox to be eradicated worldwide.[3]

The story didn't quite end there, however. In recent years, rumors about the original vaccine coming from horses rather than cows have caused scientists to rethink the centuries-old story. Jenner himself had suspected that cowpox originated from horsepox and sometimes used material directly obtained from horses to inoculate against smallpox.

Not a lot is known about horsepox, and the virus seems to have become extinct, although it possibly remains circulating in an unknown reservoir. Studies mapping its genome show it to be very similar to some old vaccinia strains, bolstering the hypothesis that the vaccine could have been derived from horses. In a letter to the editor published in the *New England Journal of Medicine* in 2017, researchers said they discovered vials of smallpox vaccines from the nineteenth century that contained the horsepox virus.[4] And to add another layer of puzzlement, both horsepox and cowpox may originally have been rodent poxviruses that only occasionally infected livestock. At least one company today is revisiting a live, modified horsepox virus to develop a COVID vaccine, modifying it to target the COVID spike protein.

Dr. Larry Brilliant, a visionary epidemiologist, technologist, and philanthropist, had the privilege of seeing the last case of smallpox in the world during his crusade to end the "speckled monster" scourge in the 1970s while working in collaboration with the WHO. He is one of our generation's most decorated and celebrated public health experts with a sharp eye on ending pandemics as CEO of Pandefense Advisory and chair of the advisory board of the nongovernmental organization Ending Pandemics. Over the years, he has become a friend, and our communication is often in Hindi, which he knows quite well from all the time he spent in India. While he didn't choose his last name, I tell him that it suits him very well. It was while working in India, the last place on Earth where smallpox persisted, that Brilliant came across a young girl named Rahima Banu who had contracted the virus in October of 1975 at the age of two and survived. She was the last case in an unbroken chain of transmission of killer smallpox that went all the way back to Pharaoh Ramses and beyond, probably 10,000 years.[5] "Billions of people died of smallpox," Brilliant reminds me. At one stage of the virus's treacherous march across Europe, it was the single biggest cause of death, killing 400,000 every year. In the Americas, it ravaged Native Americans and led to the collapse of entire cultures. It slaughtered around 30 percent of those who contracted it, leaving a third of survivors blind and almost all who did not die scarred for life. Medical historians have even suggested that we owe part of our longevity today — a doubling of life expectancy between 1920 and 2020 — to the smallpox vaccine and eradication of the menace through activism and vaccination campaigns.[6]

"The miracle is that the people came together and did it [ended the pandemic]. The magic is the science, but the miracle is

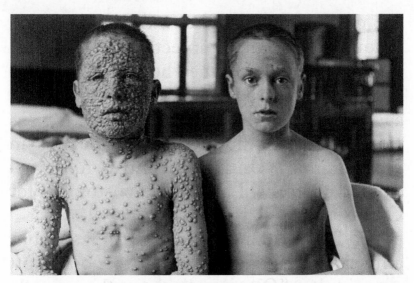

This photograph of two thirteen-year-old boys — one vaccinated and one not — was taken in the early 1900s by Dr. Allan Warner of the Isolation Hospital at Leicester in the United Kingdom. It was part of a series of photographs by Warner that were published in the Atlas of Clinical Medicine, Surgery, and Pathology *in 1901. Warner photographed a number of smallpox patients in order to study the disease. Both boys had been infected by the same smallpox source on the same day, but only one (on the right) had received a vaccination in infancy. Note that while the boy on the left is in the fully pustular stage, the boy on the right has had only two spots, which have aborted and have already scabbed. Apparently, the parents of the boy on the left were swept up by anti-vaccination fervor when they decided not to inoculate their child.* SOURCE: THE JENNER TRUST. THE PHOTO IS PART OF A COLLECTION HOUSED AT DR. JENNER'S HOUSE, MUSEUM AND GARDEN IN GLOUCESTERSHIRE, ENGLAND. FOR MORE, GO TO JENNERMUSEUM.COM.

the people," Brilliant says. Smallpox was a unique germ in that it infected only humans. It didn't have any other hosts, so exterminating it was easier once we had the vaccine against it. COVID, however, will be a virus we chase as it mutates and circulates in other animals. Until the world is fully vaccinated, there will always be customers for COVID.

Ask Dr. Brilliant what he thinks about anti-vaxxers and he's quick to point out, amusingly, "Oh, you mean the people against cows?" Much of the vaccine avoidance among anti-vaxxers has stemmed from the notion that the only way to be protected from an illness is to contract a bit of the illness itself. Many people fear that vaccines will cause the illness against which they protect. But that's the beauty of vaccines: They offer the protection without devastating illness. Today's vaccines also have the benefits of modern science; they are exceedingly safe and rigorously tested (even the new COVID vaccines that gained emergency use authorization were tested in clinical trials on tens of thousands of individuals first, and adverse reactions attributed to the vaccines are exceedingly rare; according to data from the CDC, you're three times more likely to get struck by lightning than die from a COVID vaccine).[7]

Brilliant loves keeping anti-vaxx propaganda lying around, especially items from more than a century ago, like the cartoon at the start of this chapter. Such ridiculousness reminds him of how there's nothing new about the anti-vaxx movement. The distrust of doctors and the government that feeds the anti-vaccination movement might be considered recent, but its roots were put down well over a century ago.[8] In the late nineteenth century, tens of thousands of people took to the streets in opposition to compulsory smallpox vaccinations. There were arrests and fines, and people were even sent to jail. Some of the rhetoric that anti-vaxxers used way back then is still employed today, but with greater force now that we have the Internet and social media platforms. People's soapboxes are bigger and their megaphones are louder. I happened to be working on a documentary about vaccine hesitancy prior to the pandemic, which my team and I fine-tuned and aired in April 2021 (interestingly, in 2019 the World Health Organization named vaccine hesitancy among the top ten threats to global health). When I spoke with Dr. Peter Hotez, a world-renowned virologist, researcher, and outspoken vaccine advocate, he called vaccines "the most powerful technology humankind has ever invented."[9] His group at Baylor College of Medicine produced one of the first SARS vaccines, and he continues to champion vaccine diplomacy — the global partnerships we must create among countries rich and poor to head off major health problems. From his perspective, the anti-vaxx movement of late gained oxygen and moved from the fringes to the mainstream around 2015. The movement was well shaped by targeted messaging, shrewd organization, and strong leadership — something that is not much seen in scientific circles, whose leaders tend to be siloed and usually silent. There is also a lot of money fueling the anti-vaccination movement in the form of books, live events, and medical products. I found it incongruous that many people will consume these products, which haven't undergone any safety or efficacy testing, but avoid vaccines, which have been through stringent and rigorous medical trials.

For far too long, scientists turned a blind eye to the antiscience folks under the thinking that by not paying attention to them, they'd go away or at least not be heard. But that has changed significantly now that the anti-vaccine community has established a following that perpetuates the disinformation. As much as we celebrate the remarkable science of these new COVID vaccines, their full utility won't be recognized until enough people take them. Science can rescue us only if we do our part.

The whole point of a vaccine is to teach the immune system what that pathogen — a virus, bacterium, fungus, or parasite — looks like. It gives the immune system a giant WANTED sign with the list of names and identifying details of the bad guys to look out for and attack if they show up. This can be done in several ways: inactivated vaccines, live-attenuated vaccines, toxoid vaccines, subunit/recombinant/conjugate vaccines, viral vector vaccines, and the newly developed messenger RNA (mRNA) vaccines.[10]

Inactivated vaccines do not contain live viruses or bacteria, but either whole killed germs or simply parts of these organisms. These microbial parts are DNA, protein, or specific molecules on the germ's surface. They allow your immune system to identify this as the enemy and obtain advance notice if that pathogen were to invade. Immune system cells then have a memory that allows them to recognize the organism when they next encounter it in order to produce

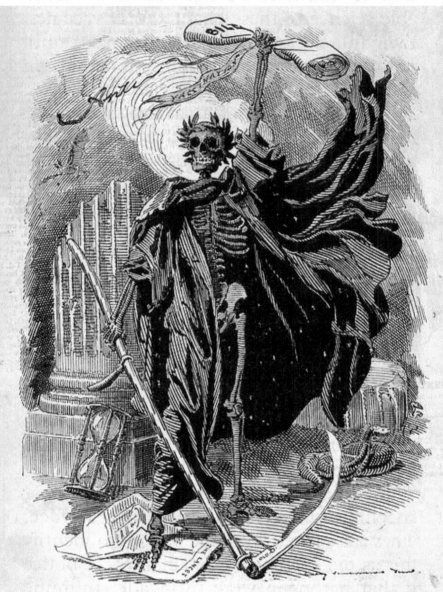

TRIUMPH OF DE-JENNER-ATION.

[The Bill for the encouragement of Small Pox awaits Third Reading in the Commons.]

1898

The title of this wood engraving by Sir E. L. Sambourne (1898) and owned by the Wellcome Collection in London is "Death as a Skeletal Figure Wielding a Scythe: Representing Fears concerning the Vaccination Act 1898, Which Removed Penalties for Not Vaccinating against Smallpox." The act had originally forced vaccination but introduced a clause allowing people to opt out for moral reasons. It was the first time "conscientious objection" was recognized in UK law. The growth of anti-vaccination sentiment reached full force in the 1890s with the National Anti-Vaccination League. The group organized protests and produced its own publications to distribute anti-vaccine propaganda. In this artwork, Death, adorned in a cloak and laurel wreath, is brandishing a roll of paper labeled "Bill" and "Anti vaccination." A coiled snake, an hourglass, and the Lancet *medical journal are scattered around the* skeletal figure. SOURCE: THE WELLCOME COLLECTION, LONDON.

antibodies to fight it. The immune cells remain circulating in your blood on guard, ready to stop an infection in its tracks if your body is later exposed to the real thing. It's armed and ready long before the invasion. Often these antibodies either don't loiter in your body for your whole lifetime or aren't enough to protect you after just one shot, which is why booster immunizations are recommended — for example, for whooping cough and rabies. Inactivated vaccines are also used to protect against hepatitis A and some types of influenza.

The smallpox vaccine was a live-attenuated vaccine. Other live-attenuated vaccines include the measles vaccine, the rotavirus vaccine, the chickenpox vaccine, and the yellow fever vaccine. A toxoid vaccine should not be confused with a "toxin." A toxoid is merely a form of vaccine that is an inactivated bacterial toxin. Examples include toxoids against diphtheria and tetanus. These types of vaccines enable the body to render the real toxin harmless if it were to show up in the future. Tetanus is exceedingly rare today (fewer than thirty cases per year occur in the United States), and most doctors have never seen a case. Tetanus is not like other infections that can spread between people. It's a spore-forming soil bacterium and is transmitted by entering an open wound. Its spore can survive on surfaces, like a rusted nail, for long periods, only to start replicating in the unsuspecting person who steps on the nail. The spore produces a toxin that causes powerful and life-threatening muscle contractions, unless, of course, the person has been vaccinated.

Like inactivated whole-cell vaccines,

subunit/recombinant/conjugate vaccines contain not live components of a pathogen but small fragments of its outer surface protein. This is what stimulates a protective immune response. Some examples of subunit/conjugate vaccines are those for hepatitis B, HPV, meningococcal disease, and some for influenza and shingles.

Viral vector vaccines use a modified version of a different virus as a means to deliver protection. For example, the Johnson & Johnson and AstraZeneca vaccines for COVID employ a harmless disabled adenovirus to convey the instructions for making antibodies. The adenovirus, which causes the common cold in activated form, is not at all related to the coronavirus but it triggers the immune system to respond without infecting the person. Viral vector vaccines have been used for Ebola outbreaks and are under study for Zika, flu, and HIV.

The new mRNA COVID vaccines represent a new class of vaccines because of their RNA technology, but the concept is the same: Introduce instructions to the body for making a protein that the immune system will tag as a bad guy so when the real bad guy shows up, the body is ready to effortlessly fight and take care of it (you probably won't even know it). I should state clearly and firmly that these mRNA vaccines do not contain the live virus that causes COVID. They contain only the code for a small portion of the virus, the spike protein. They do not affect or interact with your DNA whatsoever. In fact, mRNA never enters the nucleus of the cell, which is where our DNA is kept. The cell breaks down and gets rid of the mRNA soon after it is finished using the message.

I like to think of vaccines as language instructors: They teach the human body a new language. If you're constantly speaking in that language, such as regular exposure to the virus, the immune system gets pretty good at communicating in this new language. As the virus starts to wither away, there's less conversation in this new language, and every now and then, a refresher course may need to be given in the form of a booster shot. That quickly reminds the body how to fight the virus, especially if it has had a slight wardrobe change since the original strain.

As previously noted, viruses contain a core of genes made of DNA or RNA wrapped in a coat of proteins; in the case of COVID, the virus is RNA based. To make its now iconic spike proteins, the RNA genes of the virus make messenger RNA that then leads

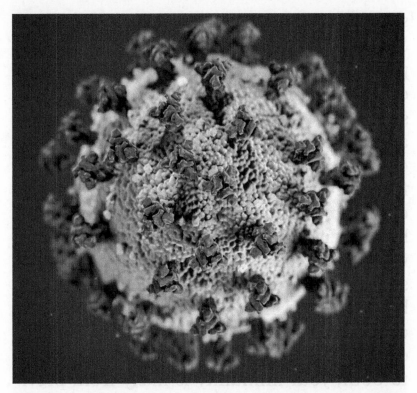

This illustration, created at the Centers for Disease Control and Prevention (CDC), reveals the ultrastructural morphology exhibited by coronaviruses. Note the spikes on the outer surface of the virus, which impart the look of a corona, or crown, surrounding the virion. SOURCE: CDC.

to the production of the proteins. An mRNA of a specific structure makes a protein of a distinct structure.[11]

Again, it is important to remember that mRNA is a message, and in your body at this moment, there are thousands of such messages being delivered. They are messages that disappear or expire quickly like a Snapchat. The vaccine is a message for one particular coronavirus protein, not the dozens of proteins that make up the virus, so there is no way the mRNA could actually lead to the creation of a virus in your own body. For this reason, the antibodies from people who are vaccinated are different from the antibodies from those who have been infected. In those who have been vaccinated, the antibodies are specific to the spike (S) protein, while those who have been infected may also show antibodies to other parts of the virus, such as the nucleocapsid (N) protein. If you have antibodies to both, your immunity is likely from previous infection.

The first steps taken to make mRNA-based vaccines did not occur on day 1 of Operation Warp Speed. It was thirty years ago that scientists began exploring the possibility.[12] The question they raised: If you know the exact structure of the mRNA that makes the critical piece of a virus's protein coat, such as the spike protein of the COVID germ, could you make that mRNA easily and quickly in a lab setting? The concept seemed simple and doable: Manufacture the mRNA that holds the recipe for a certain virus's protein coat, then inject that mRNA into someone so it travels through the bloodstream and alerts immune system cells, then confers immunity. But it turns out that the feat was not easily achieved.

We first had to learn how to modify mRNA so that it did not produce violent immune system reactions that could be deadly on their own. Once we figured that out, we next had to become proficient in encouraging human cells to not only pick up the mRNA as it passed by in the blood and produced large quantities of the critical piece of protein, but also generate antibodies to the protein. Finally, we had to learn how to enclose the mRNA inside microscopically small capsules to protect it from being destroyed by chemicals in our blood. That's a highly simplified version of the mRNA lesson plan that scientists executed as they worked to develop these new vaccines. Of course, they'd also come across some unexpected findings along the way, one of them being that mRNA vaccines trigger a stronger type of immunity than traditional vaccines. These new mRNA-based vaccines for COVID have the power to inflict a double whammy against the virus — they stimulate the immune system to make antibodies *and* immune system killer cells. That's like possessing two different kinds of ammo just in case one is not as effective.

I had the pleasure of speaking with two of the chief scientists behind the Pfizer/BioNTech mRNA vaccine that was the first to be approved for emergency use by the FDA on December 11, 2020. Of the thousands of conversations I've had while reporting on the pandemic, this may have been one of my favorites. Soon after the Chinese released the virus's genetic code in January, Drs. Uğur Şahin and Özlem Türeci got cracking thousands of miles away in their German laboratory on designing an mRNA vaccine to hit the virus. It's where they'd been studying mRNA technology for cancer research but could easily pivot to tackle this new challenge. They had all the tools at their disposal as well as the competency and capacity. Previously, no new vaccine had been developed in less than four years. The race was on, though, with a raging pandemic that could not wait at least four years.

Şahin and Türeci are a married couple with Turkish roots who founded BioNTech in Germany in 2008; their love for each other is matched by their love for science and medicine: After their wedding ceremony in 2002, they immediately went back to their lab to work. "Translating science into survival was what we shared and why at some point we decided to do this journey together of translating science into drugs and vaccines," Şahin said.

As doctors who specialize in cancer treatments, they described for me "the sense of urgency that cancer brings to people's lives." And when Şahin read an article in the *Lancet* in January about the quickly spreading coronavirus in China, his gut instinct told him that a full-blown pandemic was upon us. Vacation plans at the company were canceled and Project Lightspeed was born.

Soon after they identified several promising vaccine candidates, they needed help testing them and bringing them to market. By March, they forged a relationship with Pfizer, and that "beautiful friendship and collaboration," as they described it, resulted in the world's first effective and safe COVID vaccine. Pfizer took no federal money from Trump's Operation Warp Speed to research and develop a vaccine but did land a supply contract to provide millions of doses. It was a big gamble with no guarantees, but one that ultimately paid off.

It's important to reiterate that these new breakthrough vaccines are built on many previous breakthroughs and innovations, from biological ones like understanding the structure and function of DNA and its mRNA offspring to purely technological ones such as the ability to transmit large bundles of information (e.g., sequencing data) around the world in seconds. Şahin describes some of the biology in elegant terms, referring to mRNA as the most fundamental way to transfer knowledge to cells. He calls mRNA an intracellular information molecule — the first biomolecule in life invented by nature to enable proteins to be produced based on a grand plan mastered in the DNA. It helps to think of DNA as the hard copy information and mRNA as the soft copy of this information to tell cells what to do next. As its name implies, mRNA are truly messengers — the body's couriers.

Already, mRNA technologies have been tested to treat sickle cell disease, and they are also being tested for use against infectious agents such as Ebola, Zika virus, rabies, cytomegalovirus (CMV is a common herpes virus), and influenza. Şahin and Türeci expect the technology to revolutionize many areas of medicine, including cancer treatments and genetic diseases like cystic fibrosis, where mRNA technology could produce vital proteins that are missing in an individual. Even cancer cells make proteins that can be targeted by mRNA vaccines, though this is a more difficult challenge. For starters, not all cancers are the same. What makes curing cancer such an ambitious feat is the heterogeneity of the disease: Within a single cancerous colony of cells, for example, you have a diversity of cells with different markers. And cancers between different individuals are also unique. So imagine being able to personalize cancer treatment with an mRNA vaccine that can be designed to target those unique cancer cells. You figure out the molecular makeup of an individual's cancer, extract the information, and select the markers against which to use a custom-tailored mRNA vaccine. The versatility and speed with which you can perform this exercise using mRNA technology is breathtaking and potentially limitless.

Şahin and Türeci's success story has made them wealthy billions of dollars over, but they don't seem to have changed their lives much as a result. They continue to live with their teenage daughter in a modest apartment near their office. They don't even own a car; they ride bicycles to work. One of their star biochemists who was among the masterminds of mRNA technology, Hungarian-born researcher Katalin Karikó, also recalls the decades of adversity toiling in the lab and enduring serial demotions in academia. She and her longtime collaborator, immunologist Dr. Drew Weissman, figured out how to make the mRNA technology work. Karikó is a senior vice president at BioNTech overseeing its mRNA work now, having moved there from the University of Pennsylvania in 2013 when the school determined that she was "not of faculty quality."[13] The one thing she does struggle with today is comprehending the fact that her forty years of research are poised to change the lives of billions around the world.

Speed and versatility are important when it comes to chasing COVID with vaccines in the years ahead. Changes in the spike proteins drive the variant strains, but our vaccines can still meet the challenge. As more mutations accumulate, tweaks to the vaccines will probably be necessary, like editorial tweaks to written copy to make it stronger and tighter. But we can be well prepared for COVID's iterations with enough disease surveillance and routine sequencing to keep track of the virus's evolving characteristics. In the meantime, preventing viral transmission through vaccination is essential to contain the virus and foil its natural tendency to refashion itself.

IMMUNOLOGY 101:
THE BEAUTY OF BS AND TS

I can't cover the benefits of vaccines without dishing out some basic biology about your body's immune system. It will help you complete the picture in your head about why vaccines are so vital.

The human immune system, which is tasked with keeping you healthy in the face of bacterial, viral, fungal, parasitic, and other invaders, has two main components: the innate immune system and the adaptive immune system.[14] The innate immune system is the first line of defense. Parts of it include physical barriers like your skin and mucosal membranes, which physically stop invaders from getting in. It also includes certain cells, proteins, and chemicals that do things like create inflammation and destroy invading cells. Whereas the innate immune system is immediate and nonspecific (it tries to stop anything from entering the body), the adaptive immune system is targeted against a specific and previously recognized invader, which takes a bit longer to kick into gear.

The adaptive immune system includes a type of white blood cell, called a B cell, that patrols the body looking for bad guys. Each B cell has a unique antibody that sits on its surface and can bind to a unique antigen (the technical name for the foreign invader) and stop it from entering a host cell. When it finds and binds to a bad guy, the B cell gets activated: It copies itself and churns out antibodies, eventually creating a mega-army of neutralizers for that particular invader.

That's where antibodies come from that are created by the immune systems of people who have had COVID. Unfortunately, concerns have risen from a few studies that antibodies to this particular corona-virus can fade away pretty quickly, especially in people who have had mild cases of COVID. This has worried many researchers because if the antibody response fades quickly, we don't know how long a person who has been infected with this virus will stay protected from a new infection. This is also worrisome since we are relying on vaccines to trigger an antibody response to help protect us, and we want that protection to last a long time.

Fortunately, antibodies aren't the only weapon our adaptive immune system uses to stave off an infection. Enter the T cell. T cells, which come in three varieties, are created by the body after an infection to help with future infections from the same invader. One of those T cells helps the body remember that invader in case it comes knocking again, another hunts down and destroys infected host cells, and a third helps out in other ways.

After you get an mRNA COVID vaccine, cells in your arm muscle pick up those tiny, fatty droplets that contain the mRNA. The cells start producing a spike protein, which makes your body think its muscle cells are infected with the coronavirus.[15] Because of this, your body will try to fight off the simulated infection in the cells with its innate immune system. That's what causes some of the inflammation that people experience — the sore arms, fevers, and/or muscle aches. What happens next is those cells that have replicated the COVID spike protein (RNA) are seized by immune cells that can communicate with the special cells that make antibodies. Through this exchange, antibodies specific for COVID are generated. This process takes place in your adaptive immune system.

In the case of other vaccines made with DNA, the outcome is the same: a delivery of instructions to the immune system to wake up to the COVID virus. The method of delivery, however, is not directly from an mRNA strand. Instead, a modified adenovirus is used. Adenoviruses are common viruses that typically cause colds or flu-like symptoms. Scientists can deactivate these adenoviruses so they act as vehicles for transporting the coronavirus spike protein gene into cells, without the ability to replicate inside those cells (translation: they do not cause infection). After the vaccine goes into a person's arm, the adenoviruses bump into cells and latch onto proteins on their surface. The cell engulfs the virus in a bubble and pulls it inside. Once inside, the adenovirus breaks away from the bubble and travels to the nucleus where the cell's DNA is stored. There, the adenovirus inserts its DNA into the nucleus so those spike protein instructions can be read by the cell and copied into an mRNA that leaves the nucleus and begins assembling spike proteins. In turn, the proliferation of spike proteins alerts the immune system and promotes the same production of COVID-specific antibodies and activated B and T cells.

Many of these vaccines, both mRNA and DNA based, require two doses spaced a few weeks apart. People who feel lousy after the second dose for a day or so can thank their immune systems for showing signs that the vaccine is working. The first dose mimics an infection and organizes the troops, albeit weakly. The second shot riles up the troops and tells them this is serious, turbocharging your immunity against the virus to full capacity. People who experience a reaction after the first shot may attribute that to a previous exposure to COVID whether they were aware of it or not. But to be clear: People who have already gone through a natural infection with COVID should still receive the vaccine because it will boost their overall response to a possible future infection. Examples of other vaccines that require multiple doses include the measles-mumps-rubella (MMR) vaccine, vaccines against hepatitis A and hepatitis B, and the shingles vaccine.

As the United States ramped up its rollout of vaccines in spring 2021, I paid a visit to Pfizer's manufacturing plant in Kalamazoo, Michigan, and met with the president of global supply, Mike McDermott. Millions of doses were being manufactured every week, and they were on track to get to 2 billion doses by the end of the year.[16] Their ability to scale up production tenfold has been a remarkable feat of awesome technology combined with improvements and innovations along the way. Although Pfizer could repurpose some of its equipment, most of what I saw did not exist the previous year. Before Pfizer even knew if they had a product that worked and long before clinical trials would start, the company had spent hundreds of millions of dollars — almost $2 billion by the time I was there.

Before Pfizer decided on its final vaccine candidate, it was looking into four options, which meant that McDermott and his team had to be ready to go in any direction. He described the dilemma to me as like trying to plan an amazing dessert but without knowing what you're supposed to make. So you start buying up all the raw ingredients to make a cake or brownies, but also a pie or ice cream. "Filling up this pantry," McDermott quipped, "was quite, quite expensive."

For McDermott and his team, one of the biggest hurdles that had the possibility of slowing things down was the availability of those raw materials and specifically lipids, the fatty substance that safely houses the mRNA until it can get to our cells. Lipid nanoparticles had not yet been used in a large commercial product, making lipid suppliers in high demand all of a sudden. Pfizer worked closely with these suppliers to build more lipid capacity and also began making lipids on-site.

Ultimately, the successful production of so many vaccines came down to a gizmo the size of a quarter. "The heart of this whole machine," McDermott showed me, "is what's called an impingement jet mixer," he said as he twirled it around his fingers. The impingement jet mixer, also known as the tea stirrer, works by simply pumping lipids in one side and mRNA in the other, forcing them together with around 400 pounds of pressure. That's what creates the lipid nanoparticle that is essentially the vaccine. These aren't just any lipids; the company had to design the right combination of four different lipids that would not only protect the mRNA on the way to cells but then release the mRNA once it gets there. And while the process of creating lipid nanoparticles is not new, McDermott said the challenge was scaling up this process. The first time he saw the impingement jet mixer, McDermott thought, *You can't be serious?* His confidence was low. He could not fathom pushing billions of doses through the device. But they eventually solved that problem by replicating the quarter-sized mixers and putting technology in place to ensure efficiency. It was McDermott's moonshot.

"As a kid, my dad worked for NASA," McDermott told me. "He was lucky enough to be in mission control in Houston when Neil Armstrong stepped on the moon right at that amazing moment. I could never imagine having a moment like that in my life. Right? Like, what's the odds that something like that would ever happen again?"

When he shipped his first batch of vaccines from the facility on December 13, 2020, McDermott felt the moonshot moment rush over him.

On my tour of the plant, I saw the warehouse, the vaccine production area, and the freezer farm — the place where they store the vaccine at ultracold −80 degrees Celsius (your freezer is about −20 degrees Celsius, or −4 degrees Fahrenheit) while they're waiting to be tested. All of the purity testing, processing, and paperwork takes about thirty days, and then the vials are ready to ship. Now the race is on to keep production going and develop new variant-specific vaccines as necessary. I remember talking about the newly authorized vaccines on television one evening in December 2020. The anchor just asked me to reflect on the moment, which wasn't something I had really thought much about. I had been reporting more intently on the trial process, interpreting the data and manufacturing. After a second, I said, "The story of these vaccines will be told for generations to come," with the same reverence we have spoken of remarkable public health leaps of the past. Even beyond this pandemic, the pace of medical innovation has forever been changed by what happened this year.

It's like the story of Roger Bannister and the four-minute mile. In 1956, he was the first person in history to break that record, which many believed wasn't possible for a human to do. Shortly after that, however, someone else ran even faster, and now there are teenagers who can do it. Bannister was amazing for being first, but his legacy is more about showing us what is possible. The same is true of these vaccines.

My hope is that as people learn more about how these vaccines work and came into being, they will be universally embraced for the modern marvels they are rather than feared or, worse, shunned. As a doctor, I am often asked, "What would you do?" in a certain situation. I think it is a fair question because it requires me to put all the pieces of information together — big and small, clinical trial results and anecdotal case reports — and then make a decision. That is what I always do for my own patients and my family as well. As the only doctor in the family, it was my role long before I was ever reporting on television. And after doing all that homework, I elected to receive the vaccine and recommended it to my parents. As soon as my kids' age group opened up for vaccination, I made sure they got their shots too to protect them and help reduce overall viral spread. As I have often said about childhood vaccines, it's not just because I love my kids that I vaccinated them. It's because I love your kids as well.[17]

TOP 10 MYTHS DEBUNKED[18]

Myth: The vaccine will make me infertile, increase my risk for cancer and dementia, and who knows what else.

Truth: The COVID vaccine does not affect fertility. The COVID vaccine was falsely linked to infertility because of the syncytin-1 protein I defined earlier that is an important component of the placenta in mammals. It shares similar genetic instructions with part of the spike of the new coronavirus. If the vaccine causes the body to make antibodies against syncytin-1, it was argued, it might also cause the body to attack and reject the protein in the human placenta, making women infertile. The similarities are not remotely close enough to make a match though. It's like two people with phone numbers that both include the number 5. They share a digit, but you couldn't dial one number to reach the other person.[19] Plus, if the infertility theory were true, we'd see a shift in fertility statistics among the tens of millions of people who've been infected or vaccinated. During the Pfizer vaccine trials, twenty-three women volunteers involved in the study became pregnant, and the only one who suffered a pregnancy loss had received not the actual vaccine but a placebo.

Myth: The vaccine will change my DNA.

Truth: Without an understanding of biochemistry, it's easy to think that injecting genetic material into the body will somehow mix with our DNA and change it. But that is not the case (and if it were, imagine what we'd be able to accomplish!). You are not a GMO after being vaccinated. Nor are these vaccines "gene therapy," another subject entirely unrelated to COVID. First, the mRNA vaccines act as messengers to cells without ever entering their nucleus. They hand-deliver a recipe for making those spike proteins, and then they are destroyed by the cell (they shoot the messenger). Viral vector vaccines that use DNA (e.g., adenovirus) do go into the cell's nucleus, but they do not integrate with your own DNA. These vaccines, which have fifty years of history, act like delivery shuttles to serve up the genes for making the same antigen COVID spike protein. Unlike retroviruses such as HIV, wild-type adenoviruses do not carry the enzymatic machinery necessary for integration into the host cell's DNA. That's exactly what makes them good vaccine platforms for infectious diseases.

Myth: People who take these new vaccines are guinea pigs. Researchers rushed the development of the COVID vaccine, so its effectiveness and safety cannot be trusted.

Truth: The vaccines were authorized quickly in part because red tape was cut, not corners. As noted, the mRNA vaccines were created with a method that has been in development for decades. The companies could start the vaccine development process early in the pandemic because they were at the ready to deploy this technology. The more traditional vaccines also came into being from decades of experience. The vaccine developers didn't skip any testing steps, but conducted some of the steps simultaneously to gather, and share, data faster. These vaccine endeavors had plenty of resources, as governments invested in research or paid for vaccines in advance, or both. Social media helped companies find and engage study volunteers, and millions of people have now proven the vaccines' success. Because COVID is so contagious and widespread, it did not take long to see if the vaccine worked for the participants who were vaccinated.

Myth: I never get flu shots because they give me the flu. Why would I get a COVID vaccine when it will also make me sick, from side effects to the illness itself?

Truth: None of the vaccines for COVID can give you the disease. The spike protein that stimulates your immune system to recognize and fight the virus does not cause infection of any sort. Any side effects from the vaccine are related to the immune system waking up and doing its job. And with regard to flu, you cannot contract influenza from a flu shot. People who feel sick from a flu shot can either blame their own immune system kicking into gear or blame an illness they contracted naturally before the flu shot had enough time to work. Similarly, these COVID vaccines also need time to work. Upon inoculation, you're not instantly immune to the virus. You reach full vaccination status two weeks after a single-dose vaccine like the J&J one, or two weeks after the second mRNA shot. And you don't want to miss that second mRNA shot. Although you do have some immunity a couple of weeks after the first jab, slightly over 50 percent, you need the second jab to fill up your immunity cup to the 90 per-cent–plus level of protection. When people become COVID positive and develop symp-toms soon after vaccination, they may have contracted the virus before the vaccine has time to deploy, or fall into the small percent-age of people who don't achieve enough protection. And contrary to other reports, once vaccinated, you do not shed virus because of the vaccine.

Myth: I've already had COVID, so why bother with the vaccine? I'm immune natu-rally. And I have allergies, so . . .

Truth: It is true that your previous infection has offered you protective antibodies and likely revved up other parts of your immune system as well. Still, there may be a benefit to getting vaccinated because the vaccine appears to offer better protection against the emerging variants and stronger protection overall. While we haven't seen significant reinfection rates in the United States, other countries with emerging variants such as Brazil have been hit quite hard. Even people with severe allergies, including ones that require them to carry an EpiPen, can safely receive the vaccine and are encouraged to do so under special supervision in a health care setting. For people who have had COVID and go on to experience long-haul symptoms, getting vaccinated appears to significantly diminish or totally eliminate those symptoms in many patients.

Myth: The vaccines contain questionable substances, some of which could be used to monitor or control me — maybe even turn me into a zombie.

Truth: Contrary to misinformation swirling online about what's in these vaccines, they do not contain any suspicious ingredients or "toxins" as some say. They do not contain any dubious material, such as implants, microchips, or tracking devices. In addition to the main COVID-killing ingredient found in their genetic instructions, they also contain a support staff of fats, salts, and a small amount of sugar. And they were not developed using fetal tissue.

Myth: Once I'm vaccinated, I'm bulletproof and can fully return to normal life.

Truth: Once vaccinated, you are very well protected against severe illness, break-through infections, and the possibility you could still be contagious. Still, we need to practice infection prevention precautions until a large percentage of the country — and world — is immunized. In areas of the world where there is still significant viral transmission, while unlikely, the odds are higher you could become an unwitting carrier, even after being vaccinated. It's as simple as that. Mask wearing may be recommended in certain situations and environments until enough people are immunized, which will likely coincide with a very low rate of new cases — when the average daily rate of people testing positive in a given area is much less than 5 percent. That number reflects a time when this coronavirus response could go from mitigation to containment. We could finally get our arms around this and test, trace, and isolate the last few embers of the disease. Even if the virus is out there at that point, it would be far less consequential.

Myth: Everyone around me has already been vaccinated, and the pandemic is under control, so why bother getting vaccinated? Can't I stay unvaccinated in the herd?

Truth: We do not know what level of immunity in the community confers "herd" immunity. The exact percentage required for community immunity for COVID is a moving target. Herd immunity for measles, which is highly contagious, requires around 95 percent of the population to be immunized. In spring 2021, based on the contagiousness of the virus, the target is close to 75 percent for COVID. New variants, however, continually change the community immunity equation. The more contagious the virus becomes, the higher the percentage of people that need to get vaccinated. On top of that, the distribution of vaccines on a global scale is uneven, so pockets of unvaccinated communities may remain to fuel variants ready to hop on a plane and threaten those living in vaccinated areas. The imbalance between low-income countries and high-income nations, especially those that can produce their own vaccines, will likely continue until we have equitable global access through programs such as the Vaccine Alliance (known as Gavi) and the Coalition for Epidemic Preparedness Innovations (CEPI). Unlike other products of intellectual property, vaccines are not easily reproducible by lifting patents and sharing recipes. There's an art to developing vaccines, and it takes years of experience. Moreover, it's hard to set up a new manufacturing site quickly with all the equipment, infrastructure, and vaccine ingredients, not to mention bringing in an experienced staff to produce a large number of high-quality vaccines. Finally, keep in mind that adults make up roughly 75 percent of the population in the United States, but not all adults are willing to be vaccinated, and some may choose not to vaccinate their children that make up the other 25 percent. The more we encourage vaccination across all ages, the closer we get to community immunity.

Myth: The variants are going to come get us eventually and continually outpace the vaccines. Why be the recipient of a useless vaccine? They don't even prevent infection or transmission from what I've heard.

Truth: Combating the variants starts with aggressive vaccination to prevent the virus from replicating and changing. And the vaccines are not useless even when they are weakened by a variant. They are the bullets against the virus whether they hit the middle target or otherwise disable the fitness of the virus.

With regard to infection, Dr. Redfield highlighted a counterintuitive detail to me about the virus-vaccine relationship that most people miss: Vaccines are not necessarily intended to prevent infection. What they do is modify the viral-host interaction. They tip the scales in favor of the host, making it less likely for the virus to cause disease. That means we can be vaccinated, be showered with viral particles by a nearby sneezer, and become infected. The virus can still get in, but the host is no longer a very hospitable environment, and that means the virus might not replicate as well, or enough, to cause symptoms. Powerful new strains like Delta, however, could potentially transmit from vaccinated individuals. So vaccines don't necessarily prevent infection, but they

do a much better job at dampening transmission and illness. They also, not so unim-
portantly, are nearly 100 percent effective at
keeping you from dying of the disease. Note
too that you may not necessarily have to
follow the same brand or type of vaccine for
future booster shots. A mix-and-match approach may prove to be even more effective
at protecting you.

Myth: I have a lot of underlying conditions,
including chronic inflammation, allergies,
and chemical sensitivities to a lot of environmental exposures. The vaccine is one giant
exposure I know my body can't handle.

Truth: Having underlying conditions that
can worsen and further complicate a
COVID illness is all the more reason to get
vaccinated. In fact, people with high-risk
medical conditions, including cancer, autoimmune disease, and heart conditions, are
prioritized for vaccines. The vaccine is not
an "exposure" that will exacerbate an underlying illness. For those with serious concerns
about their conditions and the potential side
effects from the vaccine, it's a good idea to
partner with a doctor to help you through
the decision. But again, we cannot confuse
serious adverse events with the expected

side effects of getting the vaccine. About 10 to 15 percent of vaccine recipients can expect to experience side effects such as headache, arm pain, fatigue, and fever. These clear up after a day or so. Again, it shows the vaccine is doing its job — preparing your immune system to fight against the coronavirus.

SLEEPING GIANTS

The oldest virus ever directly sequenced belongs to an extinct lineage of hepatitis B.[20] It came from a man likely in his mid- to late twenties who lay down to die seven thousand years ago in a valley that is now in central Germany. He was probably a farmer. Our genetic tools today managed to lift a tantalizing clue from a tooth to explain his young death: a piece of viral DNA code that infected his liver. Although hepatitis B can be prevented now with vaccines, it continues to infect hundreds of millions of people around the world and remains a major global health problem. And while it targets and infects the liver, it also enters the bloodstream and circulates through the body, winding up in bones and teeth, where it can be preserved. The WHO is leading vaccination campaigns to immunize the world against this ancient plague.

It may feel disheartening to know that we may have to live with COVID — a newly emerging plague — in our environment for the rest of our lives. But that may be the least of our worries going forward as we pull through this pandemic and prepare for another one someday. Many pathogens, some much deadlier than COVID, lie in wait for a close encounter with our kind. Viruses in particular have an advantage over other pathogens because they are not alive, so they can theoretically hide out for as long as it takes to strike when the settings are right.

Case in point: A few years ago, scientists in France awakened a gigantic, ancient virus from its 30,000-year-long slumber in Siberian permafrost that's ready to infect again.[21] Now, this virus, dubbed *Pithovirus sibericum,* only infects single-celled amoebas (whew!). But the discovery has scientists wondering what other microbes are hidden in melting permafrost awaiting another chance to find a new host. If a 30,000-year-old virus can maintain its infectious abilities, other microbes are capable of revisiting humanity in catastrophic fashion, which is to say: There may be no such thing as total eradication of a virus. Devastating diseases like smallpox could come back to haunt us if we're not careful.

The good news is that we have modern science — and the lessons we've learned — on our side.

■ ■ ■ ■

PART 2
BECOMING
PANDEMIC P.R.O.O.F.

■ ■ ■ ■

It is illusion to think that there is anything fragile about the life of the earth; surely this is the toughest membrane imaginable in the universe, opaque to probability, impermeable to death. We are the delicate part, transient and vulnerable as cilia. Nor is it a new thing for Man to invent an existence that he imagines to be above the rest of life; this has been his most consistent intellectual exertion down the millennia. As an illusion, it has never worked out to his satisfaction in the past, any more than it does today.

— *Lewis Thomas,* Lives of a Cell: Notes of a Biology Watcher, *1974*

On a single day sometime in spring 2020, I received roughly 14,000 emails — about one email every six seconds. Each time the watch on my wrist vibrated, I looked, and my brain was taken in a new direction. Ten times a minute, even when I should've been asleep. Never before in my life had I been this inundated and this busy, and that counts my chief residency in neurosurgery, when I regularly worked over a hundred hours a week. By the time I started responding to one email, several more had buzzed in, sometimes urgently requesting a response to a note I had yet to read.

My wife jokingly asked me what all the emails were about. I smiled and said I wasn't sure, but thought they had something to do with a new breed of calico cat. She asked if I happened to receive any emails about the novel coronavirus. I shook my head and said, "No. What's that?" The exchange made for therapeutic comedy relief. And I really needed it!

We have all gone through one of the most historic events in our lifetime. It has taught us a lot about ourselves, our relationships, our environment, and the planet's delicate balance. Although scientists have accurately predicted such a pandemic for decades, it still came as a surprise for many; perhaps we'd been in denial and diverted our attention to prepare for other, more immediate threats, such as terrorist attacks and cyber-security breaches. It can be hard for us humans to prepare for something not yet visible or tangible — something that neither we nor our parents have experienced before. Some of us do take the necessary steps to mitigate the consequences of natural disasters such as hurricanes because they happen with frequency and predictability. But a public health crisis on the scale of COVID? If you had been forewarned in 2010 of what could unfold a decade later, you might have been skeptical; a once-in-a-century pathogen that sweeps across the globe decimating societies and their economies seemed inconceivable.

The truth is that the chances of a pandemic happening are the same tomorrow as they were yesterday and remain today. But something important has changed immensely: our perceptions. Friends of mine outside the world of medicine and public health have received a crash course in viral dynamics, antibodies, and vaccines. These are the words spoken in different places, cultures, and languages all over the world. We have been given a painful reminder that we share the planet with organisms of all kinds, and every now and then, those organisms leave their native habitat in search of new hosts.

We will live increasingly with the threat of a germ, probably of viral origin, making a jump from another animal to a human, causing illness, accelerating in the shape of human-to-human transmission, and then hopping on an airplane, train, or boat in an unsuspecting host to wreak global havoc. The confluence of climate change, deforestation, habitat loss, human migration, mass rapid transit, and aggressive conversion of wildland for economic development paves the way for making outbreaks of disease more common and more dangerous. These are sometimes nefarious pathogens that prey on the vulnerable and take advantage of the most human of all interactions — a handshake, a hug, a kiss, that is, any interaction where we touch or share air with one another. And once these pathogens arrive, they will likely want to stay.

According to Bob Redfield, "This virus is with us probably for as long as this nation's a nation. It's not gonna disappear." The 1918 flu never left either. Its descendants are still around in the form of a more predictable seasonal flu.

But Redfield is also hopeful. We will learn how to dance — how to coexist with this virus as it changes, mutates, and responds to the pressures we put on it through vaccines and naturally occurring immunity. With every passing month as more people develop immunity and their defenses are bolstered against the virus, the kinetics of the virus will change. It's a two-way street: As we learn about the virus, the virus learns about us. As we adapt, the virus also adapts. That is the race. Build our defensive immunity before the virus learns how to breach the gate. Then tap-dance our way through a planet we cohabitate on with microbes and pathogens. A deeply religious man, Redfield still abides by a core pillar of public health: *never leave science on the shelf.* He often recalls an old lyric from an American war song: "Praise the Lord and pass the ammunition."

So what does all of this mean for next

time? Beyond having science rescue us in the form of marvelous vaccines, how do we individually inoculate ourselves from the next disastrous pathogen and keep our families safe? How do we protect our bodies, and also our minds? What are the practical lessons to follow now to protect your future health and that of loved ones? And what if there is no obvious end, and you become a long-hauler with chronic health challenges stemming from the infection? The answers to those questions — and so much more — are in this part of the book. Life ahead of us is not about vaccines only — it's about vaccines *and.*

Through hundreds of hours of my conversations with experts from all disciplines of our society, a theme emerged: As audacious as it may sound, it is possible for a society to become essentially pandemic proof. As much as we think of national security or even Internet security, pandemic security requires lots of investment, planning, and hard work, so I've taken all the wisdom I've gleaned from experts around the world to design the pandemic-proof plan, and it entails the following P.R.O.O.F. acronym:

P Plan ahead. We should never be caught off guard again.

R Rethink and rewire risk in your brain. Evaluate uncertainty and deal with unseen threats.

O Optimize health. Prime the body for pandemic proofing.

O Organize family. Learn how to live everyday life anew (with a twist).

F Fight for the future of us. Your health depends on everyone else's around the world.

Lewis Thomas was one of the world's most brilliant thinkers and writers of his era. A poet-philosopher of medicine, he was president of the Memorial Sloan-Kettering Cancer Center and dean of the medical schools at New York University and Yale, but he was most famous for his lucid essays in which he translated the mysteries of biology for ordinary people. In his classic book *The Lives of a Cell,* which won the National Book Award in 1974, he writes about our fragility as humans who live on an otherwise robust planet. This perspective dovetails with what I've often thought about: What if we humans are the virus? Think about it. The metaphor holds up: We have found a willing host in planet Earth and are using up its resources. We've been taking our host to the edge of death, but allowing her to stay alive — a shell of her former self. We have caused a fever in the form of global warming, and we have gradually shut down Earth's perimeter defenses just like a virus slowly disables the body's own immune system. We are now even starting to search for new hosts on other nearby planets like Mars. How far will we go? How can we survive?

World War C is a call to action in many ways, written with the belief that there is a right balance between humans and host — yes, the virus and humans, but also humans and Earth. The real question is: How do we continue to coexist and even thrive on Earth, protecting our planet as a gracious, giving host and also learning to live with the ongoing threat of emerging pathogens ready to strike — COVID among them?

Welcome to a better normal.

CHAPTER 5
P: PLAN AHEAD

WE SHOULD NEVER BE CAUGHT
OFF GUARD AGAIN

Across the border to our north, Dr. Bonnie Henry was among the select few in North America who was not caught off guard when the virus landed in British Columbia (BC), where she's the provincial health officer. She had already settled in and buckled her seat belt in preparation for her province's response long before anyone in the United States had a sense of what was to come. A source of vital information through her regular addresses to the public, Henry became a household name in BC — a voice of reason through her now-famous mantra to "be kind, be calm, be safe."[1] Henry has been hailed as "one of the most effective public health figures in the world" who "aced the coronavirus test."[2]

Like Debbie Birx, Henry was no novice. She'd been trained to recognize patterns in data — not just of how viruses spread but of how government agencies tend to forget the lessons learned after each outbreak. Also like Birx, Henry had her own hard-won experience she could rely on to inform her efforts to contain and mitigate the virus's spread. British Columbia was fertile ground for the virus to flourish; it is close to Washington State, where some of North America's first cases erupted, and its large population often travels back and forth to China, where the outbreak began.

But BC didn't get clobbered, at least not initially. Under Henry's leadership, the province took decisive action the second week of January 2020 and effectively communicated to people what they needed to do to stay safe, along with the reasons and the means to do it. Let me repeat those three ingredients of the effective response: *communicate what to do, why you are doing it, and how we will help you get it done.* For example, for those who were dealing with an exposure or infection in the family, she sent her team to their homes to assist in their isolation and ensure their basic needs were met — that they had food, that the children were cared for, that the dogs were walked, and that everyone had their medications. "And then we could focus on the recalcitrant," Henry told me with a smile.

I don't want to suggest this was easy sailing for Henry. She had to convince the government to spend money and advocate massive changes in behavior that included closing schools and bars, isolating the infected, and enforcing strict social distancing. As in parts of the United States, Henry met with opposition and defiance toward some of her stay-at-home measures. Her early public warnings about expecting to "see cases soon" were also met with disbelief and anger. The premonition even struck a nerve with her superior, the deputy minister of health. To build trust with people she served, however, she knew that being forthright and open was essential despite the dire situation and the disruption to life that was about to occur. As Dr. Henry's predictions proved increasingly prescient, her relentless efforts won out. From the first time she heard about an "atypical pneumonia" emerging in China, she was also extra cautious about something few had initially considered: confidentiality. British Columbia is home to many people of Asian descent, and as in the United States, anti-Asian racism and hate crimes have been on the rise since the beginning of the pandemic. In British Columbia, this was especially true in the pandemic's early stages when cases were linked solely to China and people were calling it "the China virus" or "Wuhan flu." Anticipating that infected citizens would be targeted unfairly and discriminated against by neighbors, Henry demanded discretion when teams were deployed to people's homes.

Deborah Birx and Bonnie Henry, two of the most prominent pandemic responders in the United States and Canada, share a lot in common. Both women had careers in the military (Henry grew up a military brat and became a Navy physician). Both dedicated their lives to chasing infectious diseases and preventing pandemics, often at enormous personal cost (long days, lost marriages), and long stretches spent in some of the world's hottest spots for pestilence. And both had signature styles that the media noticed — veils of femininity that camouflaged fierce, warrior spirits. Birx's scarves earned their own Instagram account, and Henry's quirky uniform shoes by Canadian designer John Fluevog spawned a limited edition "Dr. Henry" shoe in support of the fight against COVID (with 100 percent of presale profits going to support British Columbia's food bank). The Vancouver Canucks added Henry's name to their playoff T-shirts, and the province's First Nations bestowed an honorary new name on her: *Gyatsit sa ap dii'm,* which means "one who is calm among us."[3] In mainstream circles, she became known as the great communicator, soothing British Columbians' feelings of anxiety and disconnection. She has no children of her own but came across as maternal and comforting, which was exactly what people craved. In a way, every member of her community was her child.

Henry's thirty-year medical career prepared her well for the COVID war. She'd been a female fleet medical officer tending to a thousand men at sea, a family doctor at an urban San Diego clinic, an epidemiologist setting up quarantines for families exposed to Ebola in Uganda, and the operational leader of Toronto's response to the lethal SARS outbreak in 2003. The SARS outbreak was a lasting lesson for her — and her country. When a young man entered an emergency room with a strange, tuberculosis-like disease on March 7, 2003, Henry was sent to figure it out. Truth is, she already had her suspicions because she was paying attention to something most people had been ignoring: the emerging epidemic in Hong Kong. She had raised the

alarm weeks earlier about the distant outbreak and warned it could arrive in her
country any day; she spotted the signs of a
mounting pandemic taking flight. But her
requests that hospital physicians be on alert
for severe cases of influenza — particularly
in otherwise healthy people — were ignored.
And so, tragically and predictably, before
anyone knew what was wrong, the young
man's infection quickly spread through the
emergency department. He became known
as Case A; his mother had carried the bug
back from Hong Kong and had died in their
home two days before. Henry got to work
and immediately put in place plans to
contain Canada's SARS outbreak. In the
end, SARS killed forty-four in Toronto,
many of them linked to the initial hospital.
So at the turn of the new year in 2020,
when she once again heard noise about a
serious respiratory infection spreading
rapidly in Wuhan that wasn't identifiable,
Henry's ears pricked up. This was definitely
unusual and "worrisome"; to her, it sounded
like the beginning of a pandemic. Even
though it was ten weeks before the WHO
would follow suit and officially declare one,
Henry already knew the "son of SARS" had
been born. And now it was all about responding appropriately.

It was during her time tracing Ebola outbreaks in Uganda for the WHO that she learned another critical and often over-looked component of an effective response. After explaining what people needed to do and why, she had to go the extra steps to make sure it could actually be done and explain how to do it. For example, an effec-tive quarantine would work only if food and housing were prioritized along with frequent communication. Punitive measures like restrictive mandates and fining people who defied public health measures were deem-phasized, a lesson she carried out in 2020. Instead, she championed the three Cs: confidence, competence, and compassion. Henry earned her confidence and compe-tence in all those years responding to outbreaks.

Compassion comes in handy when trying to manage people's behavior through a crisis. In a crisis, people are anxious, and that's normal. She had to strike the right balance between fraying people's nerves with bad, apocalyptic news and telling the truth of the unfolding crisis so they could prepare and keep themselves and their loved ones safe. "For many issues in public health," Henry says, "knowing when to push — and when to keep the solution in your back pocket until just the right political and societal moment — is a critical skill."

It was a superpower for Henry, but it was still a challenge to get the balance exactly right. As cases in her community rose, memories of the fears, grief, sadness, and anger that she'd faced during the SARS outbreak all came flooding back. She fought back tears while delivering public announcements. She knew that kindness and compassion, understanding others' suffering, would be the best way she and her community could overcome the pandemic.

Dr. Henry also addressed a question I have often thought about in my own reporting: Do we underestimate people's capacity to understand complex things? I have concluded that people like hearing from scientists and doctors on the front lines. They like understanding our assumptions and our ability to concede there is not yet a clearcut answer. The audience can handle the words *I don't know* and forgive the lack of a conclusion as long as you are honest and transparent about it. People often like to see the process of how scientists think through a problem and search for solutions. Medical television dramas from *Chicago Hope* to *Grey's Anatomy* actually do this really well, embracing the fallibility and dilemmas of doctors and nurses while also celebrating their lifesaving powers. But in the real world, we probably don't share our background thinking enough and instead deliver sound bites that lack nuance and are not always useful to the public. After twenty years of medical reporting, I have come to believe that we should not underestimate people's intelligence and thirst for details even when those details are hard to grasp. When it comes to their own health or that of their loved ones, people can appreciate complexity.

A fundamental question that remains to be answered is whether COVID will become endemic much like HIV — always around and always changing. Or whether it will more closely follow in the footsteps of other respiratory scourges like tuberculosis and flu, both of which are ailments that annually strike millions around the globe. The truth is, even after a hundred years, we still have a lot to learn about flu. We don't take the time to create early-warning systems for when flu begins to circulate in communities and there are subsequent surges, to identify and screen many cases of flu, "but maybe we should in the future," Birx said to me. "Maybe that should have been part of our pandemic preparedness — that we really do understand how many flu cases there are, that we really do diagnose all of them. Is there an asymptomatic component to flu? Are there children in school that we think are spreading flu? Are they really the core spread of flu? You know, sometimes we have the technology, but we don't utilize it."

It is clear now that we need to build a sophisticated monitoring system that not only tells us the extent of spread but detects new variants as they start to emerge. Understanding the moment of spread from animals to humans is more critical than we have previously appreciated. Imagine the number of lives that could have been saved if we had surveillance to identify the first intrusions of these pathogens from wild animal to human. I have always found it so remarkable that humans have such a hard time detecting microbial menaces, given the existential threat they may pose. Think about it. Germs cannot be seen, smelled, heard, tasted, felt, or even suspected. As a result, our evolutionarily ancient "lizard brain" is defenseless against these microbes. Our brain makes us afraid of the dark, jump at loud noises (what's called your acoustic startle reflex), and have an innate fear of falling, but it demands a high-tech surveillance system to tell us when something is amiss in our pathogenic environment. Some fears must be *learned.* Unlike those other fears we're born with for basic survival, we're not programmed to notice nefarious, microscopic threats. This necessitates two critical actions going forward.

1. Testing routinely to know where the virus is and where it's spreading. Testing is our "eyes" on the virus.
2. Performing genetic analyses on the virus as it mutates and spawns new variants or strains. Genomic sequencing is a sophisticated tracking of the evolution of the virus.

There are probably thousands of strains of the virus more transmissible and deadly than others. Scientists are studying how the disease caused by these new variants differs from the disease caused by other variants that are currently circulating, as well as how these variants may affect existing therapies, vaccines, and tests. Initially, the United States fell far behind in such high-tech surveillance as other nations like the United Kingdom sped up this important strategy. But we're catching up. New variants of COVID are found every week, with most rather innocuous, simply coming and going.

Some persist but don't become more common while others increase in the population for a while and then fizzle out. When a change in the infection pattern first emerges, it can be hard to tell what's driving the trend. Is it changes in people's behavior or changes to the virus itself? As fast as our eyes and ears can spot certain threats, a crucial lesson when it comes to pathogens is that we must create new ways to identify pathogenic threats as quickly as possible.

There was something else that Henry and Birx shared in common: a recognition that their scientific acumen would be greatly diminished if the messaging didn't properly connect with the masses. During the several hours of conversation I had with Dr. Birx, it was this point she really wanted to convey. And she shared three important lessons that we must consider going forward:

"People's perceptions are their reality."

"You can legislate behavior. You can't legislate how people think."

"We have to tackle how we talk to people, hear people, and meet them where they are. Who delivers the message is almost as important as the message itself."

This last insight was particularly moving for Birx while she was on the road. She tailored the message for her audience and to some extent even tailored herself to be the right messenger. When she was on college campuses, she played the part of scientist and grandmother, warning young people not to be so flippant about getting infected because we don't know what this will do to someone at thirty, forty, or fifty years old. (As we'll see in chapter 6, children who contract the virus today may go on to develop complications either during the acute phase of the illness or many years from now for reasons we have yet to understand.)

When Birx met with tribal nations and spoke with their leaders who were committed to bringing their community together, she was the public health epidemiologist and social psychologist who seized on their unwavering sense of unity to protect one another, understanding that they were living in multigenerational households, that they had one of the lowest life expectancies in the country, and that they could have made a million excuses for why things would not go well for them. And yet, together they rallied against every one of those excuses and made a difference. Standing in solidarity with them, Birx was frank with tribal health officials about their members' vulnerabilities: high incidence of coexisting chronic health conditions like diabetes and obesity, and underfunded, understaffed health care systems within their communities. She held roundtables to bring together local governors and tribal leaders to show them what to do to minimize the loss of life and take some of the distress out of the raging pandemic on the reservations. She also shared the evidence that following the simplest precautions of wearing masks, physical distancing, and paying attention to their health hygiene — in both public and private settings — could help overcome many of the unique challenges they faced.

For example, when she met with the Salt River Pima-Maricopa Indian Community in Arizona, she championed their #SHIELDUPSALTRIVER campaign and was gifted a face covering by the tribe's health officials that was emblazoned with the symbol representing a modified version found on an O'odham (Pima) warrior shield used in battle. Now it represents the tribe's fight against the virus. Make no mistake, however: Native Americans have been disproportionately affected by the virus compared to their white counterparts. In 2021,

President Joe Biden's $1.9 trillion COVID relief package provides $31 billion for tribal nations and Indigenous people so they can better prepare and at last address long-standing challenges like poor health care that make them starkly vulnerable in a pandemic. Tribal nations are communities within themselves, but they are also part of our larger national community. And as much as each one of us thinks and acts on an individual basis, we must always keep our neighbors — our community — in mind.

"We must learn how to be part of a community — not separate from the community," Birx notes. That leads us to the P in P.R.O.O.F. — Prepare. There are three important steps to prepare for your future with this virus: gain perspective; find your sources of valuable and trustworthy information; and be prepared to go into pandemic mode at a moment's notice. We'll take each of these ideas in turn.

GAIN PERSPECTIVE

In retrospect, I am surprised at how quickly the world changed. I would not have imagined that the vast majority of the country and world would actually stay at home. That the air would get cleaner. That schools would so quickly go online. That restaurants, museums, and gyms would close. Telehealth went from being mostly unused to 80,000 visits in a month at Emory University Hospital in Atlanta where I work. I was surprised at the proactive efforts of organizations like the National Basketball Association to curb the spread despite the huge monetary loss. And once we began to open up again, I watched as we delicately found the right balance between being overly cautious and not being cautious enough; finding a new normal and clawing ourselves back to some semblance of "life." In chapter 7, I'll outline essentials to putting health first and practicing extreme self-care that will be helpful to paving your personal path forward, but for now, let's focus squarely on the broader perspectives.

Pandemic burnout definitely hit by 2021, a year into the event. Perhaps paradoxically, even though the world slowed down while most of us were under quasi–house arrest, we still found ourselves exhausted and unmoored. We lost track of the days as one blurred into the next. Every mental health professional I've talked to has said that rates of depression, anxiety, stress, and malaise are all up considerably from prepandemic 2019. I think every one of us has experienced some level of posttraumatic stress (PTS), whether we or a loved one developed an infection or not. In addition to the loss of life from the virus, which alone must be grieved, there have been gradations of loss across a vast spectrum: loss of jobs, businesses, and income; loss of health and sense of well-being; and loss of signature experiences and milestones in life such as graduations, weddings, vacations of a lifetime, and family reunions. The term *brain fog* became common not just for people suffering from the illness's cognitive effects but also for individuals who escaped infection but nonetheless felt the pandemic put them in a fog that would not lift. Some people told me the loneliness of social isolation was the cause: it was harder for them to stay focused or accomplish mundane tasks. And then there's the greatest stressor of all: persistent uncertainty, the loss of security, and the reduced capacity to be optimistic about the future. So how do you gain and maintain perspective in the midst of all that?

I've reported on and written extensively about the detrimental effects that stress has on the brain and body. The kind of stress brought on by the pandemic is indeed among the most toxic and mentally crippling because it checks all the boxes: it's relentless, tedious, unwelcome, unruly, and ultimately highly disruptive to our routines — particularly those that contribute to our health. No matter how toxic something is, having an end date can help you mentally prepare. But there was no calendar to follow during this pandemic. Even the most experienced people, infectious disease doctors included, were often left saying, "I don't know." When trusted authorities admit they don't know, that brutal honesty can be unnerving and invite a sense of hopelessness.

It is why perspective is a critical component of preparedness. Without a well-informed perspective, none of the other preparedness plans can fall into place. It's an active task requiring you to take stock of the present, look toward the future with resolve, and make sure you are constantly controlling the things within your power along the way. One of the best and most productive places to start is with your own body. Getting a good night's sleep, eating well, breaking a sweat regularly for your physical health but also diligently engaging with others and even developing new knowledge, hobbies, and skills for your mental health. I realize none of this is easy and that for many, those basic activities of life have been partially sidelined or abandoned during the pandemic. Some people did become fitter and happier in 2020, but my guess is the majority of people would call it the worst year of their lives. That is why proper preparation means that so many of these behaviors must be a constant in our lives — before, during, and after a future pandemic.

Nicholas Christakis is a physician and social scientist at Yale where he directs the Human Nature Lab. He is also the author of *Apollo's Arrow: The Profound and Enduring Impact of Coronavirus on the Way We Live.*[4] I admire Dr. Christakis because not only does he have immense experience as a doctor, but he also has an esteemed career as a sociologist, studying how our social behavior influences — and is influenced by — health and human biology. He looks to history to try and project our future.

According to Christakis, gaining perspective can be more easily achieved by thinking about the impact of COVID as three distinct phases: the immediate period, the intermediate period, and the post-pandemic period that he believes will realistically begin in 2024. We were still in the immediate period when we spoke, with constant mask wearing, physical distancing, and periodic business and school closures to slow the spread of the virus. Vaccines had begun to roll out, but community immunity was not expected to be reached until likely the end of 2021 or the beginning of 2022. Some of that community immunity, which marks the intermediate period of the pandemic, would also come from natural infection.

It is during the intermediate period, he told me, that we must recover not just from the biological or epidemiological impact of the virus but also from the psychological, social, and economic impact of the virus. If you look at the history of serious epidemics going back thousands of years, it takes a couple of years for a population to recover from the immediate shock of it. Millions of businesses have closed permanently. Millions of schoolchildren have missed school. Millions of people lost loved ones and were grieving. Christakis estimates that for every person who dies of the pandemic, perhaps five more who survive the infection will be seriously disabled and suffer long-term health risks, so we also need to recover from the clinical shock of the disease. Millions of people will need ongoing medical care even when the immediate mortality impact of the pandemic is behind us. So if you put all of this together, we get to the end of 2023 and the beginning of 2024 before we finally put the clinical, psychological, social, and economic impact of the virus behind us.

And then we will enter the postpandemic period. Christakis thinks that period might be similar to the roaring twenties of the twentieth century, after the 1918 influenza pandemic. Christakis tells me:

During times of plague for thousands of years, it's very typical that people become more religious when they're afraid and when there is a serious threat afoot. People also tend to avoid social contact. People stay at home. Social interaction ceases when there's a deadly germ afoot. People become more abstemious — more risk averse. They stop spending their money. All of these changes are very typical changes that are forced upon us by the spread of a deadly pathogen. But when the epidemic is finally over, all of those changes reverse. People are no longer as religious. People relentlessly seek out social opportunities in nightclubs and bars and restaurants and sporting events and political rallies and musical performances and so on. . . . People have been cooped up for a long time. People start spending their money. They become more risk tolerant. They engage in entrepreneurial activities. They've escaped death. And so they see a bigger role [for] meaning in their lives.

That's some of the good news about post-pandemic life. The other good news is that Christakis doesn't think there's going to be a fundamental long-term change in the nature of human interaction. For thousands of years, people have fled cities for rural areas during times of plague. In 2020, as the pandemic began to spread around the world, we saw this ancient pattern repeat itself. People fled cities for suburban and rural areas; some chose entirely different states. But Christakis thinks the appeal of cities, with their job opportunities, access to activities, and diversity, remains so powerful that when the plague is finally behind us in a couple of years, people will return.

Some things, however, may never fully revert, like handshaking, superfluous business travel, and going to work or school with a bad cold or flu. I will probably always have a mask handy whenever I go into a crowded situation during flu season; it's amazing to me how often we've been surrounded by people in the past who are obviously ill — sneezing, coughing — and we have just accepted it. Given the concerns about asymptomatic spread, I will be more mindful of crowd density overall. And I will opt for touchless systems and technology when interacting with communal surfaces, as well as work from home more often.

"The bleeding stops eventually" is a common phrase doctors use and one that Christakis found fitting for viewing the pandemic. COVID may have felt persistent and stubborn beyond measure, but plagues always end. I'm optimistic too that we'll see a wellspring of support for science and medicine given the impact that vaccines have made so far and the way they will continue to revolutionize our world and its overall health. I think it's possible that having seen the importance of science in confronting this worldwide threat, we may see the importance of science in other areas, such as in confronting climate change and environmental conservation. Pandemics present problems, but they can also give birth to new mind-sets and new solutions.

Full perspective during this pandemic also means fully understanding the codependency between public and economic health. The countries that had the least disruption to their economies were the ones that were able to bend the curve the quickest, even if they took more stringent measures. That has been the case in parts of Europe and Asia. I think of the body as a metaphor for the country. In the early stages of a disease (an infection in the country), the treatment may be less aggressive and of shorter duration compared to treatment at a later stage, but it has to be thorough and consistent. You probably know not to stop antibiotics or chemotherapy early because the disease won't be fully treated and the resistant cells will be left behind to repopulate. That makes it harder to treat the next time. That is what happened in the United States; we used a half measure and were surprised when the disease roared back for several more waves. We need to remember that recovery doesn't happen with a single stroke, especially in a country as diverse and heterogeneous as ours.

Although we've learned how to slow the spread through basic public health actions like mask wearing and social distancing, we have to prepare for and accept the fact that there is no switch to turn off the contagion's spread. Perspective means learning to act in the face of uncertainty, even if the threat seems far away. The key will be staying abreast of news, digesting data correctly, and making good decisions for the health and safety of our families. And all of that is dependent on how you acquire new knowledge on which to base your important decisions.

SEEK SOUND SCIENCE AND ADVICE

Peter Hotez, a vaccinologist and dean of the National School of Tropical Medicine at Baylor in Houston, Texas, has spent his career trying to end disease and poor health throughout the world, often training his efforts on poverty-related neglected diseases we don't think about in America such as leishmaniasis, Chagas, and schistosomiasis — illnesses endemic to other parts of the world. He is one of the most accomplished academicians in infectious diseases and tropical medicine of our generation. And in many ways, he's been preparing for this pandemic for four decades. His background includes a BA from Yale, PhD from Rockefeller University, and MD from Cornell. He's fondly been called the "pan man" throughout the pandemic for his panoramic view of not only the biology and science of it all but also the political framework in which we've experienced this event. His team started studying coronaviruses a decade ago when most people hadn't even heard of them. He manufactured a SARS-1 vaccine and came close to a MERS vaccine, two feats that gave him a head start for developing a vaccine for COVID when its sequence came along.

Like me, he has witnessed firsthand the devastating effects that certain diseases can have on peoples and nations. There is no question that pandemic-level ailments are "the most destabilizing force" on the planet, he says. He urges us to stop thinking of disease, COVID included, as only a health issue. For him, it's also a root cause of global poverty and insecurities of all other kinds — from food to financial — that ultimately affect individuals no matter where they live. From his perspective, what caused the failures in America's COVID response were things that scientists aren't typically taught to think about during our training: war, political collapse, urbanization, climate change, and, of course, an aggressive antiscience movement. "It's a wake-up call about how we need to re-envision medical education to train physicians to think more broadly than we do now," Hotez told me.

Medical education has to include education about how people will react and behave when under siege from a disease because that is ultimately a big part of ending it. And, as it turns out, that behavior is fairly predictable. A skim of Nobel Prize–winning author Albert Camus's existential classic *The Plague* from 1947 tells of a fictional outbreak of bubonic plague in the French Algerian city of Oran shortly after World War II.[5] It tells the story of a pestilence in a more modern setting with postwar technologies like telephones and cars, and its details are stunningly prescient: contagion, denialism, quarantine, untreatable illness, more denialism, a cratering economy, citizens cowering in their homes, and "frontline workers" willing to sacrifice themselves for their neighbors. "Mothers and children, wives, husbands and lovers, who had imagined a few days earlier that they were embarking on a temporary separation . . . found themselves abruptly and irremediably divided," he writes. He also states what we've all come to learn: "Everybody knows that pestilences have a way of recurring in the world, yet somehow we find it hard to believe in ones that crash down on our heads from a blue sky. There have been as many plagues as wars in history; yet always plagues and wars take people equally by surprise." Nostalgia becomes a dominant emotion. We long for living in any time but the present: "The feeling of exile — that sensation of a void within which never left us, that irrational longing to hark back to the past or else to speed up the march of time . . . those keen shafts of memory that stung like fire."

Dr. Hotez took a beating at the height of the pandemic for speaking candidly about the unfolding crisis while promoting public health measures and defending vaccines. He has been an enemy of the anti-vaccine lobby ever since he wrote a book a few years ago about his daughter with autism titled, pointedly, *Vaccines Did Not Cause Rachel's Autism.* At one point during 2020, a legislator in the Texan government called his scientific work in developing vaccines a self-serving "sorcery," accusing him of being in the drug industry's pocket. That did not deter him from making many public appearances in all forms of media to push back against the misinformation campaigns about the power and safety of vaccines and to promote data-driven science because he knew what was at stake. "The vaccine ecosystem is very fragile," Hotez says. "It doesn't take much for even a good vaccine to be voted off the island if the public perception is against it." Hotez believes that antiscience is one of the biggest threats to humanity, on par with a nuclear weapon: "Antiscience is right up there with things that we build a lot of infrastructure to wall off, like nuclear proliferation, global terrorism, and cyberattacks. We need to do the same with antiscience. We have to treat it just as seriously, and do something about the anti-vaccine groups beyond just amplifying the (science-based) message."

For a long time, Hotez and others believed that responding to the anti-vaccine movement would only fuel it. Over the past decade, his attitude has changed. Anti-vaccine rhetoric is a threat to public health that demands very focused attention and an aggressive response, he told me. This entails robust pro-vaccine education in schools, through mass media, and public service campaigns. As things stand, pro-vaccine knowledge is often buried on government websites. Hotez argues there should be increased funding for health departments to combat rampant misinformation and legislation to make it harder for people to skip crucial shots and harder still for social media platforms to promote anti-vaxx messaging.

Over the past decade, we have learned that the best weapon against vaccine hesitancy is not advertising from politicians, celebrities, public health doctors, our favorite news media outlets, or even athletes. The most powerful couriers to promote vaccines are the very people in our own social circles who get vaccinated and share their positive experience. If that sounds familiar, it's because it reflects a common mantra: share; don't shame. The more people we have vaccinated, the more normal vaccination becomes. A virtuous circle of confidence develops as anti-vaxx stances are denormalized. Here is another way to look at it: Much in the way we normalized taking our shoes off at airports before getting on a plane in the wake of the 9/11 attacks, we need to normalize vaccination now because we cannot afford to have little outbreaks in our community that threaten lives. Think of it as creating cognitive antibodies to beat back against the disinformation.

Even if the virus continuously surprises us, human behavior can be disturbingly predictable. In 2018, Dr. Hotez and his colleagues correctly predicted seven locations across the country where measles was most likely to emerge. A year later, there were small outbreaks in those areas, culminating in a larger outbreak when ultimately more than a thousand individual cases of measles were confirmed in thirty-one states. Measles is one of the most contagious germs ever to roam the planet, but it also has an easy and effective antidote through a vaccine. If I had to guess where hot spots for COVID will emerge in the future, I'd say the same places where Hotez predicted measles outbreaks: places where vaccine hesitancy runs high.

Hotez and I agree that how we promote and market science — from vaccines to lifestyle medicine — will become key to inoculating ourselves against future pandemics. The private sector has leveraged the power of target marketing for decades. It's time we carry that marketing genius over to the public health sector. It is a worthy challenge to make high-quality public health and medical knowledge as engaging and available as sports or fashion.

We live in an information-saturated world that offers special powers and perils. As much as the media can inform and educate, it can equally disinform and mislead, especially in a digital age. To be sure, misinformation refers to information that is false or out of context, whereas disinformation is a subset of misinformation that is deliberately created or spread with the intent to mislead or deceive people. And there's been plenty of both to go around throughout the pandemic. It's relatively easy to spot bad information when it comes from dubious sources, but when you hear people in your own circle of friends and colleagues make questionable or even outrageous and dangerous claims, it's harder to fight back. What do you say? How do you respond to challenge their thinking while preserving the relationship?

When I encounter someone with an absurd claim, I first ask where the person got that information. Nine times out of ten, the invariable answer is, "I heard it from so-and-so," or "I read that somewhere on-line," but more often than not, the person usually cannot recall exactly where the information came from. When we encounter questionable or outright false information, we must challenge it respectfully with evidence-based explanations and sources, couching our language in compassion and empathy. It means we must do our own homework and not fall into the trap of propagating falsehoods.

Here are some ways to check for false information and promote digital literacy, courtesy of Tara Kirk Sell, PhD, a senior scholar at the Johns Hopkins Center for Health Security who works on pandemic preparedness and response:

- Use Internet-based tools and services that can provide an unbiased assessment of source credibility.

- Verify the information with other news sources or trusted people in your network, or cross-reference any factual statements or recommendations with the best information available.
- Scrutinize the social media account, URL, or layout that might suggest lack of editorial oversight.
- Watch out for messages that are designed to appeal to emotions.
- Become more aware of how disinformation campaigns work.
- Think twice about the personal biases that may lead you to bad information.

A few taps of the keyboard can send you to reliable sources or down the rabbit hole toward unreliable ones. The goal is to visit reputable sites that post fact-checked, credible information vetted by experts. This is especially important when it comes to matters of health and medicine.

The best medical journal search engines that do not require a subscription are pubmed.gov (an online archive of medical journal articles maintained by the US National Institutes of Health's National Library of Medicine); sciencedirect.com and its sibling, springerlink; the Cochrane

Library at cochranelibrary.com; and Google Scholar at scholar.google.com, a great secondary search engine to use after your initial search. The databases accessed by these search engines include Embase (owned by Elsevier), MedLine, and Med-LinePlus and cover millions of peer-reviewed studies from around the world. I often tell people to put the same degree of rigor into researching these topics as you would for a new school you are considering for your child. Do your homework, and take the extra beat to verify what you are learning. In chapter 8, I'll give you some tips on how to have conversations with people who don't take the COVID threat seriously or who don't want to follow public health measures and recommendations.

AT A MOMENT'S NOTICE

Indiana Jones–like virus hunter and epidemiologist Nathan Wolfe, whom I introduced in part 1, says that while we'll continue to face threats of pandemics after COVID, our perception has forever changed. That shift in perspective is a good one. "We live in a world with such scientific capacity but flawed human psychology," he reminds me. And the flawed human psychology that interrupted our response is, thankfully, getting retrained with this new, forced perspective. This shift will allow us to respond more swiftly, especially in the early days of the next pandemic when prompt action can have greater impact.

Wolfe believes that change in perspective coupled with the fact that COVID has rallied the private sector will better position our response next time. It's a big change compared to ten years ago, when Wolfe appeared on the world's stages alongside business leaders, trying to convince them that the commercial sector had seriously underestimated the risk of epidemics. On a Prepare for a Pandemic panel in 2010 at the World Economic Forum in Davos, Switzerland, which attracts the world's leaders in business, academic, and political arenas, Wolfe faced an audience where 60 percent of CEOs believed the threat of a global outbreak was real but only 20 percent had an emergency plan in place. That same year, he'd been invited to a cruise industry conference but could not convince executives that his disease surveillance company, Metabiota, could help them avoid the pandemonium of an epidemic. Nobody was paying attention.[6]

On December 31, 2019, Wolfe's CEO at his company, Nita Madhav, was at a family wedding in Portland, Oregon, when word of a virus in Wuhan, China, reached her. An epidemiologist by training, Madhav had taken the helm at Metabiota earlier that summer after four years leading the infectious disease data science team and, before that, spending a decade modeling catastrophes. Her goal as CEO, with a team of epidemiologists, data scientists, programmers, actuaries, and social scientists, was to build the most comprehensive pandemic model possible. They started by turning to history and amassing all the data on major disease outbreaks since the 1918 flu among 188 countries and eventually developed what they called the Epidemic Preparedness Index. The model allowed one to create the criteria around a hypothetical virus such as its geographic birthplace, transmissibility, and how easily it could harm or kill people. It then showed various scenarios of how it could spread around the world. These insights can help companies respond, including pharmaceutical companies seeking information for treatment rollouts and manufacturers who need to know how an outbreak would affect their supply chain. Metabiota's system was elegant and innovative, but its most challenging and elusive factor in the model was calculating people's fear. The economic consequences of a pandemic were a complicated interplay of both society's response and the virus's behavior.

Thus was born the Sentiment Index, or what one of its designers at the company who'd studied how human beings perceive and respond to risk called "a catalog of dread."[7] The index could churn out a score from 0 to 100 based on how frightening the public would find a given pathogen. Then that number could help determine the possible financial disruptions and losses from an outbreak as businesses closed and major projects were put on hold. Madhav and her team, including Wolfe, also looked at the broader economic consequences of pandemics to figure out which societal interventions equated with what's called the *cost per death prevented*. They found that "measures that decreased person-to-person contact, including social distancing, quarantine, and school closures, had the greatest cost per death prevented, most likely because of the amount of economic disruption caused by those measures," they wrote in a chapter for the World Bank's 2018 third edition of *Disease Control Priorities*.[8]

A year later, Madhav and her team would find themselves living inside their own model's projections. On New Year's Day 2020, Madhav tried to gather data to make predictions on the outbreak, but it was difficult because no one was panicking. There was no response to measure yet. By the third week in January, the tone had radically shifted and everyone scrambled. Ben Oppenheim, head of the product team and a political scientist at Metabiota, said they had done so much to predict every aspect of a pandemic that when it actually happened in 2020, it felt like the team was reliving a well-told story. It was déjà vu.

According to Wolfe, it comes back to the new perspective the world has gained through this pandemic. The combination of heightened awareness in both the public and private sectors, he says, will be key to our future. It is about harnessing the unforgiving reality the virus has had on our conscience. COVID is persuasive, and its tools include killing people around the world, devastating economies and government budgets, and causing massive unemployment. The key to our survival will be to not forget.

5 STOCKPILING GOODS FOR YOUR PANDEMIC PREP KIT

High-quality masks. Remember the three Fs: fabric, filters, and fit. Some of the most effective masks have two tightly woven layers of outer material with a filter material sandwiched in the middle. You can use surgical mask material or even a piece of a vacuum bag as a filter between two pieces of fabric. According to research done by a group of engineers at Virginia Tech that includes some of the world's leading aerosol scientists, you don't necessarily need an N95 medical mask to stay safe from coronavirus, although that is the gold standard.[9] A high-quality, properly fitted cloth mask does a good job of filtering viral particles; a well-fitting fabric mask with a third filter layer can stop 74 to 90 percent of risky particles. Remember to have smaller masks on hand for children.

Soap, cleaning supplies, and hand sanitizer with at least 60 percent alcohol. Note that bleach has a shelf-life of about six months. A virus like COVID is most vulnerable to plain soap and water because it is encased in a fatty lipid layer. Picture a greasy pan: Would you have better luck cleaning that with soap or a bleach wipe?

Although the risk of surface transmission of COVID is low, keep indoor surfaces clean because pathogens such as norovirus and the flu spread more easily on surfaces.

Basic medical supplies like over-the-counter medicines (e.g., Tylenol, Advil, aspirin) and prescription drugs for thirty days. Have an emergency kit that includes a thermometer and pulse oximeter that measures how much oxygen is in your blood. If there is an outbreak in your community, you may not be able to leave the house to visit the pharmacy. Don't forget to think about medications for pets and other members of your household.

Personal health and hygiene basics like toothpaste, shampoo, body wash, deodorant, and feminine products. If you have a baby, stock up on diapers and wipes. Aim for an extra month's supply.

Shelf-stable and frozen food products. If you have to stay at home and avoid grocery shopping, a supply of nonperishable food will come in handy. Store pasta, canned tuna and salmon, frozen fruits and vegetables, dried beans and lentils, nut butters, soups and broths, and perhaps dessert like dark chocolate.

BE AT THE READY

On the northeastern coastline of Japan, in a forested hillside below the village of Aneyoshi, sits a stone tablet — an obelisk-like stone carved with a warning: "Remember the calamity of the great tsunamis. Do not build any homes below this point." It was placed there after a devastating tsunami hit the area in 1933, and its warning saved the tiny village of eleven households nearly eighty years later in 2011 when another tsunami landed whose waves stopped just 300 feet from the stone. Hundreds of these so-called tsunami stones, some more than six centuries old, dot the coast of Japan.

When the last wave of the coronavirus recedes, what kind of guide stone will exist for future generations? As I previously mentioned, America lacked experience with SARS and MERS to push us to rapidly respond to this pandemic. Unlike our CDC, which initially failed to protect us from threats to our health, safety, and security, the CDCs in South Korea and Taiwan helped those countries act swiftly against COVID. The Taiwan Centers for Disease Control immediately activated the Central

Epidemic Command Center and imposed home quarantines, border restrictions, a face mask distribution system, and other preventive measures. The CDCs in Taiwan and South Korea set in motion rigorous detection and contact tracing, communication, and isolation.[10] Their coordinated and immediate approach explains their successes. The memory of SARS and MERS still haunted those countries and motivated them to act. Unfortunately, we suffered from a kind of collective myopia that caused us to underestimate risks, insufficiently prepare, and lack adequate protection. Federal funding shortfalls further undermined the CDC's response. Between 2002 and 2017, the CDC's core emergency preparedness funding was cut by over 30 percent, or $273 million.[11] Insufficient funding has also meant public health labs have been understaffed or shut down, which resulted in painful effects when COVID arrived.

As the United States reinvests in the CDC to turn systemic fragility into resilience, each of us on an individual basis must do our part to keep ourselves and our families safe. This means not only avoiding the virus but also avoiding the paradox of preparation, which refers to how preventive measures can intuitively seem like a waste of time both before and after the fact. Most of us don't stop brushing our teeth because the dentist didn't find any cavities at our last checkup, and we continue to buckle our seat belts when we're in a moving vehicle even though we may not have experienced an accident recently. But with larger events with impacts more difficult to gauge, as is the case with COVID, spurring people to action can be hard. As a society, we have not been willing to invest in pandemic preparedness the way we do for defense even though this is also a threat. Remember that, according to Robert Kadlec, who spent decades developing disaster response plans, the cost to prepare for a pandemic would be a few dollars per citizen — about $30, or the cost of a couple movie tickets. We could have vaccine platforms ready to roll, virus hunters like Wolfe in the field, robust surveillance, and a strong public health infrastructure. None of that seemed important until it became the only thing that is important.

Whether it's a pandemic or our own personal health, what inspires us to do the things up front so we don't have to pay more later? What encourages us to eat healthy foods and move more today to avoid heart disease or cancer tomorrow? When I posed that same question to Dr. Kadlec, he looked at me with watery eyes and said, regretfully, "I guess it takes something like this," referring to the gravity of COVID. "I guess it takes hundreds of thousands of people dying to say, *Oh, yeah. Next time we should be better prepared.*" His response reminded me of the stories of addiction I have covered in the past. Some addicts have to hit rock bottom to finally emerge from the depths of despair. This is our own story of addiction. *Fake it until you make it. I'm going to get lucky. This is a problem that affects other people; it doesn't affect me.* And then, one day it does.

Years ago, I had a conversation with my wife about getting lightning rods for our house. She thought the guy was charging too much money and it wasn't clear that we would ever really need them. So if we never needed it, then *any* money we spent would be too much. I understood that point of view, but two things came to mind. First is the perspective of having insurance. You often have to invest in things to protect yourself against hypotheticals that may never happen. It can be a tough decision, but if you are ever in a situation where you use an item like a lightning rod, that money is the best you'll ever spend in your life. And there is also something else less perceptible, but no less important: Those lightning rods or other protective devices offer confidence and calm. When there's a lightning storm, we are much more assured that our house isn't going to burn down. That sort of anxiety reduction is a difficult thing on which to put a price. The point is that investing in prevention cannot be measured just in terms of whether the disease happened or didn't happen. It can also be measured in peace of mind, which is priceless.

For example, few people have trouble appreciating the purpose of public education. It's a clear and concrete social program designed to improve our lives. Results are measured by test scores, graduation rates, college admission rates, employment status, and so on. Public health accomplishments, however, are not evaluated by tangible metrics. Success is defined by what is *prevented* rather than what is produced.[12] This creates an odd dynamic in our calculating minds. When public health programs work, they work invisibly, and what we cannot see, we take for granted. You can't really celebrate avoiding a disease you hardly knew existed. That makes it easy for shortsighted individuals, including politicians and leaders, to deny long-term realities. And that is what they typically do.

There are also ancillary benefits of preparedness other than tools to fight a specific disease. Part of being prepared for a pandemic could mean significant investments in universal vaccines — not just a vaccine for this coronavirus but for any other coronavirus. Not just for one flu virus but for any other flu virus. In fact, scientists are currently studying how we can develop a "pan-vaccine" that will cover all coronaviruses and influenza strains. Kadlec reminded me of the investments we made when we sent a human to the moon. What was a real benefit of that other than the fact that we could say we did it? Well, a lot. Technologies like GPS came out of that, as did intraoperative navigation technology, food safety control methods, and satellite imagery.

In Greece, the Museum of the City of Volos serves to raise awareness about disasters. Originally built to house general information about the region, including facts about earthquakes and floods from the 1950s, this smart, modern museum has recently aimed its focus on promoting disaster risk awareness. It worked with disaster preparedness experts and civil authorities to identify and reach at-risk groups, develop cultural memory games, and play a more visible role in the life of the city. Now, in the wake of COVID, it acts as a case study in how organizations can help preserve collective memory about risk. We all want future generations to be in the best position to deal with the next inevitable pandemic. And knowing how to evaluate risk constantly is tantamount to that positioning.

CHAPTER 6
R: RETHINK AND REWIRE
RISK IN YOUR BRAIN

EVALUATE UNCERTAINTY AND
DEAL WITH UNSEEN THREATS

From the moment you wake up in the morning, your brain makes an untold number of decisions. Most of them occur subconsciously. In the seconds it takes for you to read this sentence, your brain will have fired off a miraculous number of electrical signals to keep you alive — breathing, moving, feeling, listening, interpreting visual cues, digesting, pumping blood, and thinking. Some of the information zipping through your billions of neurons is traveling faster than the speed of a race car. The human brain is a remarkable organ, an evolutionary marvel. Scientists often describe it as the most complex thing we have ever discovered; one of the discoverers of DNA went so far as to call it "the last and grandest biological frontier."[1] It is arguably the most enigmatic 3.3 pounds of tissue in our universe.

Every time I operate on the brain, I am in awe at this interwoven bundle of tissue that sculpts who we are and the way we experience the world. Every joy, pain, love, sorrow, worry, and fear we have is somehow embedded in there. It is your brain that allows you to adapt to environments, tell time, figure out space, know up from down, hot from cold, and wet from dry. It is the ultimate record keeper of our story. It even whispers dreams to us when we sleep. It is the commander in chief of all your other organ systems.

Perhaps most intriguing is the way the brain assesses risk because more than anyone or anything else in your life, your brain wants to keep you safe. Our very highly tuned sensory systems act as perimeter defenses, constantly scanning the environment for threats. And then, through a sophisticated data management system, the brain integrates incoming new information and cross-references it against old memories. It is then that the brain tells the body to act, and fast. Think of this as our gut instinct, relying on images, sounds, even feelings that can be processed swiftly. A baseball whizzing toward your head. Duck. An aggressive animal with sharp teeth. Run.

A bitter taste in your food: a possible toxin. Spit.

But what if a threat is truly invisible, and effortlessly evades our senses? (Fans of *The Princess Bride* will know the ideal poison is iocane powder: "odorless, tasteless, dissolves instantly in liquid.") And what if there is no memory of it on which to draw, given we have never encountered such a threat before? Something truly novel. It would be the absolute worst-case test of our ability to assess a risk. It would be like flying blind with no automated guidance system in place. And yet this is what we have asked of our brains since the start of this pandemic. Every time we stepped outside our home, had a casual interaction with a friend, or simply breathed in someone else's air, our brain tried to assess risk, and failed. COVID-19 is in many ways the perfect unseen enemy.

Over the past year, just about every call I received, as well as every discussion around our own dinner table, was a version of the same thing: What is the risk of a particular activity? Given that I was reporting on the pandemic, people often turned to me to help fill in the information their own brains could not compute. I usually recommended they err on the side of caution, staying home as much as possible, not visiting older or other vulnerable family members, and generally physically distancing from potential exposures. It was the same philosophy I told my teenage daughter when teaching her to drive. Slow down when driving around a blind corner, because you simply don't know what lies on the other side. You definitely don't want to accelerate. Truth is, though, my brain was at the same disadvantage as everyone else's. And I fully recognized the trade-offs — the significant risks to not engaging with the outside world. Our three daughters, ages fourteen, twelve, and ten at the beginning of the pandemic, had an understandable desire to be with their friends and immersed in a sea of humanity. At that age, social interaction is particularly necessary for their psychological growth. One of the most difficult times for me personally was finding my oldest daughter silently sobbing into her pillow. "I really have no idea," she responded when I asked what was wrong. Then she suddenly sat up and clung to me for the longest hug we have ever had. She was desperate for physical and emotional touch.

Yes, they love their parents, but my girls wanted out of the house, and there was a tangible risk to keeping them locked down.

I remember staring at my wife across the dinner table on many summer evenings and repeating a version of what my daughter had said to me: "I just don't know." For a guy they always counted on to have the best information, the answers didn't come easily.

So over the past year, I created my own way of understanding and assessing risk during a pandemic or any similar threat that is both invisible and novel. It is by no means perfect and it must be highly flexible, able to change as the threat evolves. More than anything else, though, it must start with an understanding of the individual who is evaluating the risk. While none of us have a memory of this virus, given that it is novel, we do have a baseline tolerance for risk overall, and that tolerance is perhaps the truest reflection of who we are and what we value.

YOUR OWN RISK TOLERANCE

In February 2020, my friend and colleague Jake Tapper called me one day to talk about a possible trip he was considering for his family over their upcoming spring break. One of his children has asthma, and so they asked their pediatrician about the risks. At the time, there were around a dozen new confirmed cases of COVID in the country, and he relayed to me that the doctor had told them there was "probably around a 0.1 percent chance of his son having a significant problem." Before I could respond, Jake then said, "So, of course, we decided to cancel the trip." As a doctor myself, my guess was the pediatrician was probably trying to allay his anxiety by citing such a small number, but for the Tapper family, it represented enough of a risk to pull back on their travel plans. Spending time on a beach wasn't worth the one in a thousand chance something could go dramatically wrong.

On another occasion, I was in the middle of a series of Zoom calls with school administrators during summer 2020. I was working on a story about school reopenings and trying to get a better idea of the plans they were putting in place. At one point, I cited some early data coming out of Wuhan suggesting that the virus had a case fatality rate of around 0.5 percent. There was a long pause, and then a superintendent said, "Whoa . . . 0.5 percent. That means 1 in 200 people will die? That is really concerning. We need to really take care and protect ourselves." Later on that same day, another person responded to the same data: "So, 0.5 percent. I guess that means we are 99.5 percent good, then, right?" A completely different response. (I mentioned these percentages much earlier in the book but now let's tease this further apart within the context of how people can make such divergent interpretations.)

It was an illuminating series of discussions that reminded me that while people may hear the same objective data, they interpret those data very differently. For many people who were able to stay home through the pandemic, even a small risk was too much. For frontline and essential workers, who had no choice but to show up, the risk tolerance could be much higher. We saw that play out in different ways throughout the pandemic in the United States. And as we started to evaluate risk tolerance across cultures, the differences became even more pronounced.

WHAT WE VALUE

I once did a story about an international group of researchers who came together from the University of British Columbia, MIT's Media Lab, Harvard University, and the Toulouse School of Economics in France to evaluate the concept of risk from an intriguing perspective: teaching the artificial intelligence of self-driving cars how to make a split-second decision when there is no way to avoid a fatality.[2] How would a car determine which person or group of people should be "sacrificed"? Science fiction fans will immediately recognize Asimov's law: A robot cannot kill or harm a human through action or inaction. But what if there's no choice? What if the brakes fail, and there is no scenario where the autonomous vehicle can save everyone?

If it sounds familiar, it's because it is a version of the classic ethical thought experiment known as the trolley problem: Five people are tied to a trolley track with a car bearing down on them. You can throw a switch redirecting the car to another track to which only one person is tied. What do you do: Take responsibility for the death of one person or allow five others to die by doing nothing? In a further iteration of the problem, the five people can be saved only if you physically push a fat man onto the track to stop the car with his body.

The more recent study, dubbed the Moral Machine experiment, launched in 2016 and allowed more than 2 million people around the world to play a game that showed preferences for sparing or, conversely, sacrificing different types of lives. It generated nearly 40 million decisions in ten languages, becoming the largest crowd-sourced ethical study worldwide. People who played the Moral Machine game were shown two images, each depicting an out-of-control car driving into a different group of people (or, in some of the images, a cat or a dog). For example, the game might tell you that if you let the car plow ahead, it will kill three little girls and two adult men. But if you swerve to the right, the car will instead kill two elderly men, two elderly women, and a young woman. Which way to swerve? Who would you kill? I found myself playing it at the kitchen counter one day, and soon my entire family was running the sacrifice scenarios.

Morbid indeed, but also revealing. The most likely to be saved were babies, children, and pregnant women. That wasn't surprising. Athletes and businesspeople were often saved at the expense of homeless people and overweight men. Doctors scored just below nurses. It turns out cats were most likely to be sacrificed. And here is where this thought experiment became so relevant to this pandemic: the sacrifice of the elderly. The data showed that in the hierarchy of sacrifice, old people came just behind cats and criminals! That all humans should be spared before pets seems morally correct but in this experiment, dogs were saved more often than criminals (and criminals won over cats). Almost always, the car was taught to swerve toward someone who was old, just like COVID did. Remember that early on in the pandemic, we quickly learned the disease was disproportionately killing the elderly, as we saw extended care facilities account for a third of all deaths in the United States.

It really got me thinking: What if the COVID pandemic had primarily killed young people instead of older folks? Would we have responded differently in the United States? Would our risk tolerance as a country have been lower? On the flip side, did the cultural reverence for the elderly in Asia lead to a more aggressive response there? Although a preference for sacrificing the old to save the young was found in every country during the Moral Machine experiment, the places where people showed the weakest preference for killing the old were in East Asian countries, places that also had some of the lowest death rates overall in the world.

The study unveiled a bitter truth that many of us knew in the back of our minds, even if we are reluctant to admit it: Certain deaths bother us more than others do — and what bothers you might not bother your neighbor. This is the reason to develop a risk assessment as a society that takes into account these subconscious prejudices and works to neutralize them.

And that is not the only obstacle to coming up with a rational response to a pandemic like this one. Our brain, the ultimate risk assessment tool, was at an incredible disadvantage initially because it had no previous memory of this particular threat.

YOUR BRAIN: PLAYING THE ODDS OF WHAT WE REMEMBER

When many infectious disease doctors first heard of a coronavirus from China, it immediately triggered a memory in their brain: SARS. They therefore reflexively put this new virus into a "SARS box" in their brain, anticipating the virus would spread only symptomatically and just disappear over time. That presumption ended up being a terrible mistake, putting many people in harm's way until we understood how COVID behaved.

The problem is a fundamental one in the world of neuroscience. The adult brain is not very good at accepting truly novel experiences. A fully mature brain will always scramble to fit the new experience into an existing one. Kids, in contrast, are wonderful at dealing with novel experiences because early in life, everything is new. That ability diminishes as we get older. We adults become increasingly reluctant to accept that something is truly novel, confident instead that we have seen it all before. After all, I'll ask again: When is the *last* time you experienced something for the *first* time?

Such a phenomenon — the inability to process a new experience — is something Daphna Shohamy, professor of psychology at Columbia University's Zuckerman Mind Brain Behavior Institute, has been studying for some time. She recently collaborated on a study that looked at how patients with damage to the hippocampus, the memory center of the brain, made decisions.[3] The research team asked these patients to make a series of very simple decisions like choosing between Kit Kats and M&Ms or between pretzels and potato chips — the sorts of mindless decisions we make all day long. Without fail, however, the group of people with damage to the hippocampus took two to three times as long to make these decisions as compared to those with intact memory.

According to Shohamy, this kept happening for a specific reason. Despite having no memory of these particular foods — how they tasted, whether they were satiating —

their brains struggled to come up with any evidence whatsoever that would help them make that decision. It was like the brain was in a constant loop, looking to find a single morsel of data to help guide the decision.

"Eventually, in those cases, the brain basically just makes a prediction," Shohamy tells me. While it is the most educated guess it can make, many times the brain gets it wrong. The lesson is a profound one when assessing your own risk. Trying to recall evidence or memories that don't exist will just get in the way, slow you down, and quite likely end up being incorrect. Instead, it takes clearing the mind and not letting preconceived notions hinder you that can more accurately help you evaluate the risk.

With COVID entrenched in our environment, we will now have to regularly evaluate risk and make decisions that affect not just ourselves but everyone around us — loved ones and strangers alike. Although we've been making decisions all our lives that affect others, the pandemic adds a new complication that each individual must consider like never before. The virus may mutate down a notch or two to become less virulent and deadly, but its presence will nevertheless probably be perpetual. As technology improves and we continually learn more, we will likely see improvements to indoor ventilation systems and protective measures that could make indoor spaces safer overall, but the risk will never be zero. And we may never reach that elusive herd immunity in the United States or worldwide no matter how much we try to vaccinate. The combination of vaccine hesitancy and a small percentage of people who don't respond strongly to the vaccines has compromised our ability to get there. And those who are not vaccinated for whatever reason can fuel breakthrough cases and more variants. The world will remain a patchwork quilt of populations relatively safe from the virus and populations that will experience outbreaks. We must learn to live with this virus for the rest of our lives and factor its risk into our days, a mental process that should become relatively automated just like a self-driving car that needs to make navigational decisions to prevent accidents. The first step to getting there is better understanding your brain.

REWIRE YOUR BRAIN

I'm spoiled in my brain world. I get to work with an organ that continually changes and reshapes itself — perhaps the only organ in the body that can grow better with age.

Every time you experience something new (like the pandemic), your brain slightly rewires to accommodate that new experience. Novel experiences and learning cause new dendrites to form, which are segments of brain cells that receive electrical impulses (*dendrite* literally means "treelike" because they are short-branched extensions of a nerve cell that reach out to nearby brain cells). With repeated behavior and learning, your existing dendrites become more entrenched. Both the formation of new dendrites and the reinforcement of preexisting ones are important, of course. The creation of new dendrites, even weak ones, is called *plasticity.* And it is this plasticity that can help your brain rewire itself if it is ever damaged. It is also the core ingredient for resilience, vital for building a better brain.

So as you navigate the postpandemic world and learn new things, changes happen to the synapses and dendrites: more connections are generated, while others may be weakened. The brain constantly organizes and reorganizes itself in response to your experiences, your education, the challenges you face, and the memories you make. These neural changes are reinforced with use and memory (hence the saying "What wires together fires together").

We all experienced some serious rewiring at various times throughout the pandemic as we normalized certain new behaviors like wearing a mask, keeping physically distant from others, and washing our hands a lot more frequently. For some, the rewiring made it harder to shift our habits again when COVID restrictions eased and we were told we could be maskless under many circumstances. My teenage girls, for example, adapted very quickly to wearing masks; it became second nature to them. Even as masks became increasingly unnecessary with vaccination, they still slipped the ear loops on as they walked out the door. Their younger brains encoded this new behavior more easily and more forcefully than their parents' older brains. And the ease with which our brains can perform this electrical mental "redecorating" makes us uniquely adaptable. It's just like learning to play a musical piece. If you play Beethoven's Moonlight Sonata on the piano over and over, for example, the repeated firing of certain brain cells in a certain order makes it easier to replicate this firing later. The result is that you get more adept at playing the piece effortlessly. If you stop practicing for several weeks, though, and then try to play the piece again, you may not be able to play it as skillfully as before. Your brain has already begun to "forget" what you once knew so well. The dendrites that were so clearly defined start to wither away a bit fairly quickly. Luckily, it is not difficult to read the notes even years later and build up those neural connections once again.

Similarly, we may need to mask up again in future years, for which the wiring we've established in the COVID era will come to good use. We now have that all-important memory to motivate us and switch into COVID control mode quickly. The pandemic-proofing habits we want to put into place going forward will require their own wiring, but the beauty of our brains is that they make it all possible. As much as you initially resisted public health measures to combat the pandemic, you eventually got used to it. And while you might resist new lifestyle habits in your personal prep for another pandemic, my guess is you'll soon get used to that too. Your brain, and your peace of mind, will thank you.

THE RISK SPECTRUM IN EVERYDAY LIFE

The Infectious Diseases Society of America helps determine which activities can be categorized as low, medium, and high risk when there's a pathogen to factor into daily life.[4] Of course, how that pathogen behaves and is transmitted matters. With COVID, a very tiny percentage of cases happen from viral transmission outdoors, regardless of vaccination status, making activities outside much lower in risk; the odds of transmission indoors, however, are more than eighteen times greater. Six feet may never be enough for indoor settings to be safe when it comes to COVID. A group of researchers at MIT found that the risk of being exposed to COVID indoors is as great at sixty feet as it is at six feet — even when wearing a mask.[5] This group, led by engineers and mathematicians, developed a method of calculating exposure risk to COVID in an indoor setting that factors in a variety of issues that could affect transmission, including the amount of time spent inside, air filtration and circulation, immunization, variant strains, mask use, and even respiratory activity such as breathing, eating, speaking, or singing. The fact that aerosolized virus particles can travel far and stay in the air for prolonged periods makes indoor settings all the more problematic no matter how far you are from other people. Think of it like cigarette smoke. Even if someone is smoking in a room on the other side of the house, you will eventually smell it. The lesson: outdoors trumps indoors. For future pandemics, a critical question will be whether the pathogen spreads primarily via aerosol or respiratory droplets.

As COVID vaccination status for the country increases overall, the risk threat will decrease in all categories. If you have been vaccinated for COVID, your risk of becoming seriously ill is very low. We now know your risk of becoming infected is also low as is the likelihood you will spread the virus if you do develop a breakthrough infection. The risk primarily is for unvaccinated people to spread the virus to other unvaccinated people. As Barney Graham, deputy director of the NIH vaccine research center told me, the country won't split into vaccinated and unvaccinated. Given the contagiousness of the virus, with time, the country bifurcates into vaccinated and infected unless basic public health precautions remain in place for those who aren't protected. What the science teaches us at this time is highly transmissible variants may mean masking up even if fully vaccinated.

IT'S ALL RELATIVE

The real question we all have to ask our-selves is this: What's the chance something will happen *to me*? You can have low-, medium-, and high-risk labels on various activities but still be stuck trying to figure out how they apply to you and your personal risk profile. Spending time with someone outside your household may seem low risk, but that may not be the case if that person carries the virus unknowingly and you have underlying conditions associated with worse outcomes. Risk is personal.

I have to deal with relative risk with my patients daily. In the simplest terms, risk is the chance something will happen. Relative risk of something happening is calculated when you compare the odds for two groups against each other. For example, the relative risk of developing lung cancer in smokers versus nonsmokers would be the probability of developing lung cancer for smokers divided by the probability of developing lung cancer for nonsmokers. If we hypothet-ically find that 17 percent of smokers develop lung cancer and 1 percent of non-smokers develop lung cancer, then we can calculate the relative risk of lung cancer in smokers versus nonsmokers as:

Relative risk = 17% / 1% = 17.

Thus, smokers are seventeen times more likely to develop lung cancer than nonsmokers.

An important point to remember is that the relative risk does not provide any information about the absolute risk of the event occurring, but rather the higher or lower likelihood of the event in the exposure versus the nonexposure group. *Absolute risk* is the odds of something happening over a particular period of time. For example, according to the National Cancer Institute, a woman living in the United States has an absolute risk of 12.4 percent of developing breast cancer in her lifetime. That means for every 100 women, around 12 will develop breast cancer at some point in their lives.

Bear in mind that a low chance of something happening — good or bad — does not mean that there is no chance. If the risk of a side effect developing is 1 person out of 100, that still means one person will experience that side effect. And it could be you.

When Johnson & Johnson temporarily paused its vaccine rollout due to the risk of blood clots, the media buzzed with confusing headlines. It presented a case study in how a new risk is evaluated in real time across a large population of people. In the United States, six women (out of nearly seven million vaccine recipients) developed a rare blood clotting disorder, vaccine-induced immune thrombotic thrombocytopenia (VITT), after receiving the J&J vaccine; two of them died from the condition. Naturally people panicked. These were women (maybe one man) younger than fifty years old, which made scientists wonder if gender and hormones had anything to do with it. The side effect appears to involve an immune response that differs from other types of clotting disorders and that predominantly affects women.[6]

The root of much of the anxiety may not have been the elevated risk of developing that side effect but rather simply not knowing how to put the risk into perspective. Here's the paradoxical fact: The risk of having a clotting problem from a COVID infection is far greater than the risk of having a vaccine-associated clotting problem. Without question, the vaccine dramatically reduces the risk of any of the COVID-associated blood clots.

Blood clots are extremely common, affecting 900,000 Americans a year, according to the CDC.[7] They kill an estimated 100,000 people annually. Clots in the brain are also common. About 795,000 people suffer strokes every year in the United States, according to the American Heart Association, and the group estimates 10 to 15 percent of these are in adults under the age of forty-five. Even the very specific type of clot associated with the vaccine, known as a cerebral venous sinus thrombosis, has a background rate of 5 people in 1 million in any given year.

Risk factors for ordinary blood clots include surgery, accidents, cancer treatments, hormonal birth control, smoking, and even sitting too long (prolonged sitting on long-haul flights, for instance, can substantially increase the risk for blood clots in vulnerable people). Although media reports popped up about people suffering more ordinary blood clots after having been vaccinated, it's unlikely those were caused by the vaccine. But it's hard for most people who aren't trained in medicine to know the difference.[8] Similarly, a person who unexpectedly has a massive heart attack (or gets hit by a car, for that matter) the day after getting a vaccine may think the event is linked to or even caused by the shot. We know that this is not the case.

The chances, or absolute risk, of experiencing clotting complications as a result of either the J&J vaccine or the AstraZeneca one that is based on similar technology is 1 in 1 million (about the same odds, relatively speaking, as dying in a plane crash but much lower odds than going to the ER with a pogo stick–related injury, the latter of which is entirely preventable but affects 1 in 115,300 Americans). The risk of a blood clot for a young woman taking the birth control pill is about the same as the risk of a person being struck by lightning.

I should also add that if you get a flu shot, there's a 1 in 1 million chance of developing Guillain-Barré syndrome, a rare disease that can cause paralysis. Another way to look at these relative numbers is the following: If 1 million people contract COVID, roughly 5,000 will die based on current data. If 1 million people receive the J&J vaccine, *maybe* one person will develop this specific type of blood clot in the brain, which is treatable if diagnosed early. Which side of the odds do you want to be on?

For me, it was easy. I picked the vaccine, and so did my wife, who was in the age group of women at risk. Part of her decision was also informed by the fact that we know how to treat adverse reactions to these vaccines. These conditions, from VITT to allergic reactions, are manageable and curable. Doctors know what to look for and treat accordingly.

LET'S PLAY RISK[9]

Common Risks	The Chances
Dying in a road traffic accident over fifty years of driving	1 in 85
Needing emergency treatment in the next year from an injury by a can, glass bottle, or jar	1 in 1,000
Needing emergency treatment in the next year from an injury by a bed, mattress, or pillow	1 in 2,000
Dying in any accident at home in the next year	1 in 7,100
Being hit in your home by a crashing airplane	1 in 250,000
Drowning in the bath in the next year	1 in 685,000

Throughout 2020, we didn't have enough information to put COVID into risk context. But now we have more data to make reasonable assessments about an individual's risk for contracting the virus and how that person will fare in the course of the disease based on a few variables such as age, health status, and access to care. It is true that the nature of a contagious disease means you need to not only account for your own risk but also the risk you may pose to others. Fortunately, there are ways to mitigate risk. It depends on three important factors:

What you do. What kinds of activities are you engaged in, and who is around you? What is the likelihood you're going to breathe someone else's air or others will breathe yours?

Where you are. Your location in the world locally determines your risk for exposure (e.g., indoors versus outdoors, in areas with high versus low COVID transmission, being where the majority of people around you are vaccinated or not.)

What you bring. Do you have any personal risk factors like preexisting conditions that could complicate a COVID infection?

REWRITING RISK: AVOID THE TRAPS

It is important to be aware that as your brain calculates risk throughout the day, it goes to a default emotional response based on limited or overly biased information.

Here are some competing interests that could be hampering your ability to assess risk fairly:

- *It's not going to happen to me.* This is called optimism bias, and it's one of the most basic, well-established principles in social psychology. People with optimism bias think their own risk is less than other people's risk. This type of bias is more prominent in individualistic, mostly Western societies like ours, where we prioritize personal choice and the rights of individuals (compared to collectivistic cultures, where the focus is on group goals and what's best for the group). And it explains why you'll choose to eat a cheeseburger and fries over fish and steamed broccoli. It's not that you don't believe heart disease is more associated with meals higher in saturated fat. You understand that, but you also think the risk is just higher for other people.
- *I'm in total control so I'll be okay.* When we feel in control, even if it's a false sense of control, we're less likely to be worried. Driving a car seems safer than being a passenger on a plane, but the

data make clear that is not the case. Driving long distances and making pit stops can entail more potential exposures than flying on a plane point to point. Similarly, when we follow public health advice and wear masks, wash our hands, and practice social distancing, our perceived risk of contracting the virus is lower and can make us act in a more cavalier way.

- *No one knows, so why should I worry?* Mixed messaging from the beginning of the pandemic from public health experts and other leaders has not helped create a unified front about the dangers of COVID. The messages around masks alone were divisive and confusing, giving some people permission to lessen their sense of true risk.

- *My social circles have all stayed healthy even though they haven't followed the public health measures.* This fallacy reminds me of my smoking patients who tell me they are not worried because they know someone who smoked their entire life and never developed lung cancer. They search for messages that reinforce what they want to hear. This happened even more acutely during COVID: The anxiety and strain imposed by the disease led people to huddle inside their like-minded groups and develop their own groupthink. The group, in many cases, became their identity.

- *I read that it's safe to eat indoors if the tables are spaced well enough apart.* This is another example of confirmation bias. You wanted to confirm a hope that it's fine to dine inside. So you search for the answer you want to find by typing in "safe dining indoors during COVID" on the Internet rather than "dangers to dining inside during COVID." Each of those searches will turn up radically different sources of information, and you will gravitate toward the ones that will assure you it's okay because they're aligned with what you wish the outcome to be.

- *I've been going to the grocery store and running errands for months now; it's totally safe.* Exposure therapy is real: The first trip outside your home in public following a lockdown may have stressed you out and made you anxious. But after braving public settings a few times and not getting sick, the outings lose their risky edge, and it's natural to let your guard down. Those subsequent trips seem less scary, but your risk may have been increasing as the actual COVID numbers were climbing in your area. The risk tied to running errands does not remain the same — it's dynamic with the ever-changing rates of community spread. Over the past year, I have spoken to hundreds of patients who became ill from COVID. Invariably they always said how surprised they were to actually have contracted the illness. Their minds had rewritten the risk even as the worrying evidence was there to see.

RISK GOING FORWARD

Now, more than a year into the pandemic, we know exponentially more about this disease than at the beginning. But it is still a small fraction of what we need to learn to assess risk. It is still unclear, for example, why some people breeze through their illness while someone who is similar in age and health background will be undone by it. "I want to find out how it could possibly be that the same virus that's killed more than half a million people in this country is a virus in which more than half the people don't ever get any symptoms," Fauci told me in spring 2021. It can be wildly different even for identical twins, like Kelly and Kimberly Standard, who also lived together. I spoke to the thirty-five-year-old sisters about what happened to them in spring 2020.[10]

After experiencing fever and shortness of breath that hadn't gotten better after a few days, both went to the emergency room and were diagnosed with COVID. Kelly said she had a bad feeling about the situation. "I've got high blood pressure. I'm diabetic. I have breathing problems — I'm asthmatic — and I think this virus is really going to affect me. I was thinking, *It's going to get worse,*" she told me. Like her twin, Kimberly had similar medical conditions but said she felt the "complete opposite": she wasn't really worried. "In my mind, I'm thinking, *Okay, let's get this out of the way and go home.*"

The Standard sisters were admitted to Ascension Providence Rochester Hospital in Michigan on the same day, and after that, everything changed. Kelly, who had the bad premonition, got better with treatment and was discharged; Kimberly became much worse. She was airlifted by helicopter to a different hospital where she eventually wound up on a type of life support called ECMO — extracorporeal membrane oxygenation. It's a machine that pumps and oxygenates a patient's blood outside the body. She spent about a month connected to tubes and machines, in and out of consciousness, battling for her life.

This vast difference in how Kelly and Kimberly reacted to the coronavirus surprised the twins and their doctors. There is still a significant randomness to how COVID affects certain individuals, even twins, and that makes calculating risk going forward all the more difficult.

THE 5 PERCENT RULE

As a general rule and reminder, you want to be in a setting where the positivity rate — the percentage of people who test positive for the virus — is below 5 percent. Positivity rates are a confusing concept for people, but here is a way to think about it. If you are fishing with a net and you bring up lots of fish, that probably means there are a lot more fish down there you are still missing: a high positivity rate. If you only bring up a few fish, a low positivity rate: that means you are probably catching most of them. But here's the thing: Sometimes you cannot know the positivity rate in your exact location. Or by the time you do, it's too late and you've been exposed. With that in mind, it is reassuring to know that regular testing could become the norm for this pandemic and future ones. Many at-home rapid test kits are coming on the market that will help us monitor where the virus is lurking and potentially spreading. This will help us get ahead of future outbreaks and keep infected people isolated.

Keep in mind too that community immunity is not necessarily permanent. It is based on the contagiousness of the virus at any given time. With COVID, the threshold for adequate immunity may be closer to 70 percent in the summer months when heat and humidity slow viral transmission. It may then pop back up to 80 percent in the cooler and dryer winter months, which is why it is so important to achieve high vaccination rates even as cases are dropping. As the threat of the virus ebbs and flows over the years, so too will risk factors.

DYNAMIC VIRUSES DEMAND DYNAMIC RESPONSES: PLACE YOUR BET

With a germ like smallpox, a single vaccination conferred lifetime immunity. Smallpox is a double-stranded DNA virus that lacks a known animal reservoir other than humans.

Compare that to COVID, which is a single-stranded RNA virus with a higher mutation rate and multiple animal hosts. Average mutation rates in RNA viruses are estimated to be about a hundred times higher than those for DNA viruses and up to a million times higher than their hosts'. Put simply, we cannot mutate fast enough to gain immunity against COVID and so we must accommodate it as an ever-present threat by constantly evaluating risk within the context of our lives and taking necessary precautions to prevent exposure.

One provocative way to put risk into perspective is to think like a poker player. When I spoke with psychologist, champion poker player, and author of *The Biggest Bluff* Maria Konnikova, she helped me understand how to think through the probable risks associated with different decisions as a serious poker player. It was an astonishing lesson for me. Maria first got into the world of poker out of a curiosity for trying to disentangle skill from chance. She wanted to find out: Where are the limits of control? Where are the limits of what we can and can't do? And where does variance enter into it? When does pure luck enter into it? How do you learn to tell the difference? We both agreed that life is a game of incomplete information; you never know everything, so the question then becomes: Do you try and always complete fully gathering the information first, or do you try and get really good at making decisions with the information that you have?

"I think you need to get comfortable with uncertainty," Maria told me, "and with the fact that any decision is going to be inherently probabilistic." She's right. As she reiterated to me, there's no such thing as certainty in anything in life. No such thing as 100 percent. Everything is probabilistic. If you get up to 98 percent, you're ecstatic. But two percent is a lot. One percent is a lot. All of those tiny percentages are actually huge when it comes to talking about billions of people and billions of outcomes. And as the stakes go up, those tiny percentages have to mean more. So the best you can do is to make the best decision you can with the information you have, knowing that it's never going to be perfect. "I think that quest for perfection can actually hinder us more than it can help us," Maria said. She also brought up a good point: We process risk through experience, but our experiences are not necessarily representative of actual statistical risk — they are skewed. So sometimes we will overestimate tiny risks and sometimes we'll underestimate risks that are actually much bigger simply because our personal experience has skewed us too far in one direction or another. Our personal biases get in the way. So, how can one correct for this? Enter a game of poker where, as in everyday life, there are consequences for keeping it too safe . . . and there are consequences for taking too much risk.

As Maria described it, poker is all about adjusting your strategy based on the circumstances. Sometimes it's going to pay to take more risks than you normally would, and sometimes it will pay to be more conservative. And the same strategy doesn't always work.

"If you're playing a game, especially tournament poker, where the stakes keep going up, you're going to go broke if you take too many risks. You're going to bleed chips. On the other hand, if you haven't been betting much, then when you do have a strong hand and you're ready to take the risk, everyone's going to fold. Everyone's going to be scared of you because all of a sudden you got very aggressive. If people aren't idiots, they'll realize, *Okay, you know, this person has a strong hand. I need to get out of the way.* And so you're not going to be able to maximize money even when you have good cards. . . . You need to find that magic middle."

For Maria, poker represents a risk exercise based on incomplete information, your own risk tolerance, and understanding how others will react to you in a dynamic situation. It is not a perfect metaphor, though, because the politicization of the pandemic in America was a wild card. It made it uniquely different from a game of poker, as people were more likely to identify with certain data that met their political party's thinking, even if it made it more likely you would lose money, or your own life. In a pandemic like this one, evaluating risk has also become a question of identity — whose tribe and way of thinking you subscribe to.

But politics aside, Maria's idea of placing a bet on a decision is a great way to assess your sense of risk. Put simply, the best way to understand uncertainty is to bet on it. How much are you willing to bet you're right about a certain risk, or wrong? This is a strategy borrowed from Immanuel Kant, who once used an apt analogy in the medical world where people tend to have a false sense of confidence in their doctor. Maria recalled the thought experiment well for me: Imagine you go to a doctor and the doctor looks at you and gives you a diagnosis and you leave. Now what if you actually stopped for a second and forced that doctor to put money on the diagnosis? How much would the doctor be willing to bet that the diagnosis is correct? $10? $100? $1,000? $10,000? $100,000? His marriage? His happiness? His life? Where's the line? "Something like that is an incredibly powerful corrective to overconfidence and to false certainty," Maria said. "All of a sudden, you're forced to actually ask yourself, *Wait, well, what's my basis for making this?*"

I couldn't agree more. Even among my colleagues, low-evidence data sometimes get presented with the same confidence as high-evidence data. Asking someone to bet on their prediction isn't glib — it is a way of setting the same table for everyone and adding a degree of accountability. It's such a brilliant way of looking at the world. Think about this too, which Maria posited: If everyone on social media in general had to put money down for every opinion, a lot of our armchair experts would suddenly evaporate.

Maria summed up her lesson by giving me a new mental construct to consider in my next risk-riddled decision-making process: Get into the mental habit of almost fact-checking yourself and thinking, *Okay,*

I'm about to make this decision. How much am I willing to risk? It may also help to pretend the situation involves your mother, your grandmother, your sister, your daughter, whatever it is. *What am I willing to risk? Do I think that the data support what I'm about to do, given that the person I'm seeing here might be actually someone I really love and care about?*

If we constantly go through that calculus, our risk assessment will change in a profound way.

As more of the country is vaccinated, we have seen plummeting cases, hospitalizations, and deaths. By spring 2021, most experts had finally started to sound notes of cautious optimism. With the increased population immunity and the warmer weather, which makes it harder for the virus to spread, many public health officials started recommending a loosening of the restrictions: fewer masks, more gatherings, restaurants, and travel. In our household, we have had more visitors, coffee dates, hugs, and dance parties.

No question, there is an earnest desire to return to normal. The vaccines have made us more willing to take a risk because the thinking is that the reward now clearly outweighs it. But with hundreds of millions of doses now administered by late spring 2021, some people decided this gave them a built-in reason not to get the shot, with the rationale that others were doing enough of the immunity work for the rest of us. As a result, the likelihood that enough people would have immunity, by either vaccine or previous infection, to reach herd immunity became more elusive. And without that level of immunity, there would always be the risk the virus could resurge and once again cause outbreaks. So how will that affect our return to normal? And how will it shape the level of risk you are willing to tolerate for yourself and your community?

There are plenty of reasons for continued caution: the variants, the heartbreaking outbreaks in India and Brazil, the inequitable vaccination rates across racial and political divides. But our risk assessment is now increasingly based on what the public can see: We are winning the war on COVID in the United States, and we have learned to adapt better than the virus can. That means being willing to again deploy tools such as testing, tracing, isolation, masking, and even brief, highly targeted shutdowns if they are needed.

SPECIAL NOTE FOR WOMEN

The disinformation campaigns around the safety of the COVID vaccines for women of childbearing years have been epic, with false ideas proliferating online that attract and persuade even the most educated people. Women have been told that the vaccines mess with their menstrual cycle and cause infertility, miscarriages, and death of babies being breast-fed from moms who took the jab. Another popular myth is that the vaccines have caused more deaths than the disease itself. Online groups perpetuating these false stories have thrived in unexpected places like mommy and parenting groups on Facebook, Twitter, and Instagram, even though these social media platforms have pledged to combat vaccine hesitancy and disinformation. By the time these dangerous accounts are removed, it's often too late. The information has already metastasized among scores of women who believe that the vaccines are much riskier than getting COVID. That could not be further from the truth.

Nearly two-thirds of anti-vaccination content posted on Facebook and Twitter between February 1 and March 16, 2021, was attributed to just twelve influencers, dubbed the Disinformation Dozen.[11] And what's truly shocking is that some of these individuals, many of whom are well financed, hold medical degrees — or they did until they let their licenses expire or were denied relicensure. Their fearmongering messages are as compelling as the conspiracy theorists who keep the Flat Earth Society going.

Let me be clear: The vaccines save lives, including pregnancies and babies. Pregnant women who contract COVID are at an increased risk for severe illness, premature birth, and maternal death compared to nonpregnant people. And vaccines will protect women who are years away from starting a family. My three daughters have all been vaccinated, and I plan on being a grandfather someday.

USE TECHNOLOGY

Several mobile apps and websites have been developed to communicate the risks of COVID to the public. This type of technology is here to stay and will play a much bigger role in future outbreaks. The Web-based COVID-19 Event Risk Assessment Planning Tool, developed by scientists at the Georgia Institute of Technology in Atlanta, estimates the probability that you will encounter someone with the pathogen at a

316

gathering, based on the size of the group and where the event takes place.[12] The 19 and Me calculator, developed by Mathematica, a policy research company in Princeton, New Jersey, leverages demographic and health information as well as user behaviors such as hand washing and mask use to determine relative risk of exposure, infection, and serious illness. And Johns Hopkins University's COVID-19 Mortality Risk Calculator estimates an individual's relative risk of death from COVID on the basis of his or her location, preexisting conditions, and general health status.

Obviously, these tools require the latest data and models to make accurate predictions. They also must take into consideration new science from the latest peer-reviewed literature to refine their infection models. The CDC's official app provides up-to-date news on health and COVID. The WHO dashboard, which follows the number of confirmed cases and deaths by world region and hardest-hit countries, is designed for easy viewing on a mobile device. There are also plenty of apps to help you lessen contact with others, participate in COVID research at major universities and institutions, and monitor your own health whether you're healthy or potentially infected.

One note of caution: Be careful about which apps you download and use. Through this pandemic, and future ones as well, there will be another constant: scammers. They have consistently taken advantage of the chaos caused by the virus. Some claim to offer apps to track COVID cases, but instead infect and lock your device and demand ransom. This type of crime is on the rise. Scammers will even pose as government or health officials to steal your money or personal details. Just when you're trying to lower your risk for infection and keep you and yours safe, you've opened yourself up to other risks. As digital contact tracing apps and exposure notification systems become more established, essential to these tools' success will not only be improving the technology but also protecting privacy and building trust before the next pandemic.

KIDS COMPLICATE RISK

If you're single, vaccinated, and healthy, the post-COVID world has opened up to you, and making personal decisions about where to go and whom to socialize with may not be that difficult. But for people with children, the risk-benefit analysis is more complex. Families make decisions based on their tolerance for risk, and there is more than one reasonable approach. As a father of three teen and tween girls, I know that too many kids suffered during the lockdown, isolated from their friends, activities, schools, and extended family. And for parents who've lost jobs and income, their children suffered further as a result.

Let's assess the death risk. COVID'S effect on children has been fundamentally different from its effect on adults: Pediatric deaths from COVID in the United States have been in the hundreds, not the hundreds of thousands as with adults. We didn't know this in the beginning, and keep in mind some viruses, such as H1N1, were more problematic for children compared to adults. While some kids infected with COVID have developed an inflammatory condition, it's very rare. When reports of children — mostly between the ages of three and twelve — developing a rare condition called multisystem inflammatory syndrome (MIS-C) hit the media, I took many frantic questions from parents worried about their own children's risk for this complication. The syndrome is characterized by inflammation of different body parts, including the heart, lungs, kidneys, brain, skin, eyes, or gastrointestinal organs and appears to be associated with a COVID infection in the past or present. Many children affected with MIS either didn't know they'd been infected with COVID, or only experienced mild symptoms from COVID before the problems began. And most are diagnosed with MIS long after the infection has cleared. Scientists are still trying to understand this newly emerging inflammatory syndrome but it once again underscores the importance of avoiding infection and protecting oneself through vaccination when possible. We just don't know what an individual's lifetime risk for other health conditions will be after recovering from MIS (and most do, though on rare occasions it can lead to serious complications and rarer still is MIS in adults).

Future variants could have a more severe impact on children, and the long-term effects of COVID are unclear, but overall, COVID is a negligible risk for the vast majority of kids with no underlying health issues. Families will have to weigh one set of dangers against another when choosing where to go and what to do with their children as the pandemic works itself out.

When I spoke with public health experts about COVID and kids, most were quick to point out that the risk for COVID is on par with the risk for flu, and the flu does not upend most children's lives. They go to school when the flu is circulating, though many do get flu shots. My hunch is that most kids will be vaccinated before the end of 2021. These experts highlight the risk of COVID within the context of other risks in a kid's life. About twice as many children drown in a typical year as have died from COVID over the past year, and about five times as many die in vehicle accidents. So if fully protecting children from low risks but serious harm was our top goal, we would keep kids away from pools and out of cars.

Now that we have a much clearer idea of absolute risk of COVID to children, we have to look at the relative risk. Dr. Amesh Adalja, a pandemic expert at Johns Hopkins University, reiterates, "Everything has risk."[13] In other words, acting in the best interest of children is not the same as minimizing COVID risk. COVID may dominate the minds of adults, but it should not necessarily tower over the lives of our children.

As we moved into spring and summer 2021 in the United States, it was clear that the light was increasingly on our faces, but there was still a stutter-stepping into normalcy as the trauma of the past year weighed heavily on people's minds. I understood it, but also reminded people, including my own parents, that these amazing medications and vaccines are created to not only save your life but to return your life to a more normal one. And while it is absolutely true that we have been humbled by the virus and its subsequent variants, we also know that zero risk is neither an attainable goal nor a worthy one. Humans have always had to tolerate some degree of risk to move forward, and that has not changed. Your obligation is to make sure you best understand that risk for yourselves and those around you.

Although many families may hesitate to vaccinate their young children, including those who have been infected naturally, it's imperative that we inoculate them now to protect their future health. As I've been stressing, we just don't know what this virus will do later on, and withholding vaccinations may fuel more variants that will come back to haunt all of us.

Respecting future risks is real. We advocate for the HPV vaccine in adolescents so they reduce their risk of cancer later in life, as the human papilloma virus can infect the cells of the cervix, mouth and throat, anus, penis, vulva, and vagina. HPV infections turn normal cells into abnormal cells that can lead to certain cancers over time. Like many COVID infections, HPV infections often have no symptoms and go unnoticed. But once you catch it, your lifetime risk for cancer goes up if your body does not effectively clear the virus, especially if you've contracted one of the thirteen types deemed "high-risk HPV."

In addition to keeping everyone up to date with vaccinations, one of the best things a family can do to stay as safe as possible in the future is to optimize everyone's health in the household for the post-pandemic era. It's the next step in pandemic proofing you and your family.

Chapter 7
O: Optimize Health

Prime the Body for Pandemic Proofing

Ahmad Ayyad didn't know where he was when he woke up in the delirium of his COVID illness.[1] The forty-year-old also didn't know why there was a tube down his throat, or how long it had been since he last fed his dog. And when he looked down, he barely recognized himself. Just weeks previously he'd been a 215-pound strong and chiseled athlete but was now sixty pounds lighter. "I woke up and looked at my arms, my legs, and my muscles were gone," he said. "I was kind of freaking out, like, *Where are my legs? Where did my legs go?*"

It had started with an overwhelming feeling of weakness. As someone who was managing his own restaurant and club in Washington, DC, while also working at his family's retail furniture business, Ahmad was the consummate multitasker. He also ran marathons, competed in obstacle course races, took basketball classes, and boxed. But then his entire life turned upside down. Everything was challenging and exhausting, from walking up the stairs to cooking, driving, and even talking. Soon the coughing and sneezing commenced. Eventually a high fever set in with a total loss of energy and appetite, and trouble breathing. At the urging of one of his friends, a physician assistant, he took an Uber to Sibley Memorial Hospital. The date was March 15, 2020. At the time, there had only been 529 cases of COVID-19 officially diagnosed in the United States, and Ahmad became another one of them. Like most other people who test positive, he didn't know when, where, or how he was exposed to the virus. Perhaps it was a three-day trip he had taken to visit his brother in Florida, but he wasn't at all certain. What was certain was that the virus had quickly debilitated an extremely healthy fitness buff. In addition to COVID, he tested positive for influenza. Ahmad was intubated and immediately transferred to Johns Hopkins Hospital in Baltimore, where he was put in a medically induced coma for twenty-five days. The last text he sent to his sister read, "Am I going to die?" On many nights, the doctors informed his parents that he wouldn't make it through the night. "My son is a fighter, he's not going to die," his father would reply.

Ahmad became the hospital's third COVID patient and the first to be placed on a ventilator. Defying the doctor's predictions, he survived and went home on April 22 with a blood clot in his left arm and damage to his heart and lungs. He spent the next month struggling to do anything without losing his breath. But his warrior spirit, as he described it, kept him going, and he made incremental improvements over the many months of recovery. Ahmad's experience was unusual given his fitness going into the illness, but it served as a wake-up call for anyone who didn't think the virus could be harmful to the healthy.

Nearly a year after Ahmad contracted the virus, Alber Elbaz succumbed to the disease in Paris at age fifty-nine. A self-proclaimed "priest of fashion," the Moroccan-born Israeli was one of the industry's most beloved designers.[2] My interview with him in 2014, when he was creative director of the designer house Lanvin, remains one of my favorites of all time. He said something then that's quite telling now: "Fashion is all about changes. You know, there is a saying in America, 'If it's not broken, don't fix it,' and I think that if it's not broken, fix it before it breaks."

It bears repeating: Fix it before it breaks. Anticipate. Optimize. Learn from the past. Do not forget. We have a lot of fixing to do . . . to keep from breaking again.

CHUNK, MONK, DRUNK, HUNK

Almost everyone I've talked to has some story of change through the pandemic whether for better or worse. I joked that you come out of this either with more weight on (the chunk), stronger spirituality (the monk), a greater dependence on alcohol (the drunk), or a leaner, fitter body (the hunk). And plenty of people have been a version of each of these individuals on the pandemic's long timeline. Early on during the crisis, as we grappled with unprecedented stress levels and competing impulses to manage fears and uncertainty, it was a given that sales of comfort foods and alcohol would soar. Stress has a powerful effect on what people choose to eat and drink. But this also led to people gaining unwelcome weight, inspiring many to pivot and focus on their health and immunity.

According to the International Food Information Council, one in three consumers said they ate healthier foods in 2020.[3]

Those under the age of forty-five were most likely to make healthier choices. At the same time, the eating habits of 19 percent of those surveyed became less healthy, and women were more likely than men to tip toward indulgence. More than one in five people admitted to stress eating during the pandemic, and one in four turned to comfort foods. Many individuals sought out energy boosters, with 28 percent drinking more caffeinated beverages — no doubt fueled by the increased demands of working from home and remote schooling of children. And while 22 percent drank more alcohol (total off-premise alcohol sales were up about 24 percent during the pandemic, and spirit sales surged more than 27 percent from 2019, with men and younger consumers more likely to imbibe), roughly the same amount tried to cut back on booze.

Throughout the pandemic, we've been hearing a lot about the risk factors for the most severe effects from COVID. The list of chronic underlying medical conditions for severe COVID and death is quite long and includes conditions as complex as cancer and as common as asthma. Historically, chronic health conditions have been attributed to older adults, or at least we often think of chronic ailments that way. But they increasingly strike younger and younger generations, with new studies showing that older millennials, those born between 1981 and 1988, report having been diagnosed with at least one chronic health condition.[4] These are people who just started to turn forty in 2021. Among the most common troubles reported are migraines, major depression, and asthma, followed by type 2 diabetes and hypertension. And experts agree that obesity is a primary driver for general unhealthiness.

In the United States, obesity is an epic problem, with nearly 40 percent of adults and 20 percent of kids living with it.[5] That's one in three adults and nearly one in five kids. I use the word *obesity* delicately but with good intention. The whole subject of obesity is shrouded in feelings of discomfort, and even shame, but now dangerous obesity raises the risk for all kinds of disorders and disease — among them COVID. It should be no surprise that wealthy nations, often insulated from the worst of infectious disease outbreaks, were hit disproportion-ately hard and some have blamed this partly on our obesity rates. This is a complex problem because obesity rates are not only higher in many rich countries, but they are also attributed to poor communities *within* those nations whose access to healthy nutritional choices is limited. As much as the obesity epidemic is a product of wealth and abundance, it's also the result of the absolute opposite — food deserts where bad calories dominate.

Obese patients who contract COVID are 74 percent more likely to end up in an intensive care unit and 48 percent more likely to die.[6] Among the more than 900,000 adult COVID hospitalizations that occurred in the United States between the beginning of the pandemic and November 18, 2020, nearly a third have been attributed to obesity. That's significant. Imagine those 271,800 people avoiding hospitalization entirely by not having been obese when they got infected. Have you ever wondered why obesity is such a risk factor? It's one of the questions I've probably answered the most this past year: What explains the relationship between weight and the chance of survival from infection? It's partly due to how our bodies are built.

The diaphragm is one of the major muscles that helps with breathing. Breathe in and the diaphragm contracts and the lungs expand to take in oxygen. But if you're carrying excess fat in the abdomen, it can place pressure on the diaphragm, forcing that large muscle to restrict the airflow in the lungs. After a short time, the airways in the lower lobes of the lungs collapse, making it increasingly difficult for the body to adequately oxygenate the blood coming through. Also, let's not forget that obesity is a precursor to other health conditions that add risk, including heart disease, lung disease, diabetes, an impaired immune system, chronic inflammation, and blood that's more likely to clot. Now toss in a COVID infection, and the risk increases. The mechanics of the coronavirus in the body make it especially harmful to people with a lot of extra weight. The cells that line your blood vessels and regulate blood flow, endothelial cells, can become damaged when you're infected with this virus. And the fat cells themselves may also be more susceptible to coronavirus. Remember: This virus attaches to cells in the body through the ACE2 receptor, which is a protein on the surface of many cells. It turns out that fat tissue has a high level of ACE2 receptors, thus functioning as a reservoir for the virus. In essence, the more fat you carry, the more "infected" you can become. You're more magnetic toward the virus.

All of us have a role to play in reversing the obesity trends, especially when it comes to its disproportionate impact on racial and ethnic minority groups (more on this later; at last count, Black and Latinx adults have a higher prevalence of obesity and are more likely to suffer worse outcomes from COVID). But if there's one silver lining to this pandemic, it is the intense attention shining on our general unhealthiness, forcing us to consider what we can do about it before another virus arrives. In my conversations with Dr. Bob Redfield, the former head of the CDC, he repeatedly lamented our challenges with obesity as a driving force in our dismal COVID outcomes. He brought up an interesting insight about the relationship between weight and a body's reaction to a virus like COVID: set points. It came up when I asked him about people who can't seem to shake the illness and go on to become long-haulers — patients with chronic symptoms that remain after the initial infection runs its course. Redfield discussed the idea that each person has a unique internal setting for managing the body's metabolism and its degree of inflammation.

Set point theory is often evoked in weight loss circles: There is a biological control method in each of us that actively regulates our weight toward a predetermined set number for each person.[7] The body prefers to stay within a certain range of weight, but if that set point becomes dysregulated or tinkered with because of overeating or undereating, the results are evident in weight gain or loss — and potentially create a new set point. Similarly, we each carry a baseline level of inflammation. Inflammation is the body's defense system for taking care of potential insults and injury, but when that system is constantly deploying chemical substances and keying up the immune system, it starts to go a bit haywire. Fire hoses are good for extinguishing blazes, but you wouldn't want a fire hose to stay on indefinitely.

It helps to think of your set point as a built-in thermostat that is programmed to a particular temperature. If your set point is high, such as a thermostat fixed at 80 degrees Fahrenheit, your general level of inflammation is higher than someone whose set point is lower. Although there may be some variations, a higher set point means a higher degree of temperature (inflammation). Now toss in a virus that wreaks havoc on the body's internal systems and self-regulatory processes. During the acute phase of infection, the virus first attacks organs and tissues, directly triggering a cascade of inflammation. After the virus leaves, however, the body may be left in the throes of an ongoing cytokine storm that can dial up one's inflammation set point indefinitely. This scenario has kept a lot of doctors up at night, worried their seriously ill patients would seemingly improve after the virus cleared, only to crash and die a few days later. We learned months later that President Trump's doctors had feared that might happen to him when he returned to the White House just days after being admitted for the infection.

Redfield is among many doctors who think our inflammatory set points can be adversely affected and reprogrammed by an infection like COVID, which may help explain the ongoing inflammatory storm that some infected patients suffer. The next question is: How can one deprogram and dial back that thermostat to a healthier setting? How do we prime our bodies to be ready for the next infection? Here's a good place to start: Remake your metabolism and nurture your microbiome.

REMAKE YOUR METABOLISM

Diet is a confusing topic. I don't even like to use the word *diet* and much prefer *nutrition*. For my previous book, *Keep Sharp:*

Build a Better Brain at Any Age, I spent an enormous amount of time researching and talking to nutrition experts all over the world about the "best diet" for the brain (knowing full well that what's good for the brain is good for everything else). I was surprised by a lack of consensus, with some experts promoting ketogenic diets or intermittent fasting, with others talking about the benefits of going gluten free. But one common denominator rang true across the board: Good nutrition and other lifestyle habits like regular movement (I also try to avoid the word *exercise*) and restful sleep have the power to drive down the risk of the major chronic diseases in the United States. And when it comes to good nutrition, there are styles of eating that do not have to conform to any single, restrictive "diet." In other words, you can find an ideal approach to nutrition that works with your preferences and personal needs.

We have enough evidence between outcomes in animal models, human clinical trials, and large epidemiological studies to make certain assertions with confidence. And I know that deep down, you already understand that eating muffins or doughnuts with a mochaccino every morning for breakfast probably isn't going to get you where you really need to go. Diets may seem confusing, but food isn't. Part of the solution is figuring out what really fuels you in the best way without producing digestive issues or food allergies. If you focus more on what you should eat instead of what you shouldn't eat, you will find yourself fueling up with good calories and naturally avoiding the bad ones. Food should be a source of nutrition, yes, but it should also be a source of pleasure. I go out of my dietary lane from time to time and have no guilt when I do.

The key to remaking your metabolism involves changing how you think about food in the first place. Food is at the center of a grand intersection: it can hurt, and it can heal. When we choose what to eat, we are determining what information to give our body — information for our cells and tissues all the way down to their molecular structure. For most of my life, I simply thought of food as fuel, just calories for energy, made up of micronutrients and macronutrients ("building blocks"). Over the past decade, though, I have come to understand and appreciate food as a tool for so-called *epigenetic* expression, or how your diet and genome interact. Of course, it matters what you eat, and your genes play a role in how you use and metabolize what you eat. This is why underlying genetics can factor into risk for certain conditions, like obesity and metabolic dysfunction. But rather than the chemical conversion of food to energy and body matter of classic metabolism, food is also a conditioning environment that can shape the activity of the genome and the physiology of the body.

You probably have not thought about food from that perspective before, but the foods you consume send signals from your environment to your genes. Those signals have the power to change how your genes behave, how your DNA is turned into messages for your body, and how your resulting biology and physiology operate. Because food is the one piece of information we all have to give our body every day, we have to be sure we send the right information that works with it and supports healthy pathways — not harmful or self-destructive ones.

Given the diversity in cultural practices and lifestyle habits around the world, there are many ways to approach dietary choices. It should come as no surprise that the typical Western diet — high in salt, sugar, calories, and saturated fats — is not friendly to our physiology when it's in excess. As the research concludes, a plant-based diet that is rich in a variety of fresh whole fruits and vegetables, particularly berries and green leafy vegetables, is associated with better health. I know you have heard this countless times, and you may be numb to it. I am too. But there are a few simple statistics I often share with my patients to make the point — for example, increasing fruit intake by just one serving a day has the estimated potential to reduce your risk of dying from a cardiovascular event by 8 percent, the equivalent of 60,000 fewer deaths annually in the United States and 1.6 million fewer deaths globally. And I'll add that if a mere handful of berries or a juicy apple reduces your risk of having a cardiac event by that much, it can also reduce your risk of experiencing a bad reaction to an infection like COVID. While no single food is the key to good health, a combination of healthy foods will help secure the body against assault, and it is never too early to begin. Think about it. The food you eat today can lay the groundwork for protecting your body in the future. Only 10 percent of Americans get the recommended number of fruits and vegetables a day.[8] More than a third of us eat fast food daily, and at least one meal a day comes from a pizza box or a drive-through.

So in the age of pandemic preparedness, what does eating well look like? It's focused, and with renewed purpose. Make no mistake: Every smart microdecision you make to nourish yourself is part of the plan to make you pandemic proof. From a fundamental standpoint, it means eating real food — not popping pills and supplements. Not to my surprise, supplement sales surged during the pandemic, with multivitamin sales increasing by double digits as people prioritized health and wellness. By fall 2020, vitamin and supplement use had increased by 28 percent in the United States and by 25 percent worldwide since the start of the pandemic. The demand for vitamins D and C and zinc also spiked when news hit that these ingredients might help fight a COVID infection and "boost" immunity. Trouble is, we don't have evidence that any specific supplement or vitamin fortifies the immune system or offers an advantage when fighting an infection like COVID. That doesn't mean they aren't helpful; it's just that we don't have the evidence. In the interim, remember the old adage: Absence of evidence is not evidence of absence. Maybe these nutrients are helpful, but we just aren't sure.

One thing that researchers do agree on is that the best way to obtain these nutrients is through food, when you get the active ingredient and the constellation of micronutrients that help the active ingredients do their job. While we all like the idea of a pill with the micronutrients neatly packaged in one swallow, that approach is not effective and not really possible. That bottle with broccoli on the label doesn't really have broccoli in a pill. The evidence shows that micronutrients such as vitamins and minerals offer the greatest benefit when consumed as part of a balanced diet because all those other components in healthy food work with the micronutrients to do their job better. Think of this as an entourage effect. While there may be some star players, they don't work as well without the entourage of other ingredients. For example, getting your B vitamins from eggs and your omega-3 fatty acids from fish always beats taking vitamins and supplements alone.

While effectiveness is challenging to prove when it comes to supplements, I believe we do have an obligation to make certain something is safe. And for the record, the supplement colloidal silver, which has been marketed as a COVID treatment, is neither safe nor effective for treating any disease. From the last day of January in 2020, the day the White House declared a public health emergency, until the end of July, the FDA and the Federal Trade Commission (FTC) sent 106 joint warning letters to supplement producers for selling products with fraudulent claims of treating or preventing COVID.[9] During the same period, the FTC separately issued 62 warning letters, and the Department of Justice obtained injunctions against three supplement producers for selling products that made claims of treating serious diseases like COVID.

I realize that changing your diet in an effort to optimize your health will take some time — and it should. Most of us have a general idea of what's good for us, what we like and don't like, and even what our own superfoods are. I kept a food journal a few years ago to figure out what worked best for me. Turns out fermented foods like pickles are my secret weapon. I snack on them to boost my productivity and energy. Find what works for you, and make it part of your routine. Reducing your intake of refined sugars and flours, artificially sweetened foods and beverages, fast food meals, processed meats, highly salty foods, and sweets is no longer a gentle suggestion; it is a mandate. Watch your portions. Prepare more meals at home where you're in control over the salt, sugar, and fat content that can hide stealthily in packaged meals or in restaurant food. (For a list of basic guidelines to follow, see *Keep Sharp.*)

In the wake of this pandemic, we will need to analyze how we nourish ourselves at a deeper level than we have ever done in the past. This past year has reminded us that we shouldn't only focus on avoiding heart disease or diabetes. We should instead have a thorough understanding of how our food can minimize our vulnerability to pathogens we haven't even yet identified.

In preparing for the next pandemic, we also need to consider the role of the microbiome — the gut's internal "friendly" germ factory that actually plays mightily into our immunity. Let's go there next.

IMMUNE BOOSTERS DO NOT EXIST

Despite slick advertising by marketers of "immune booster" products, such as those that fill the largely unregulated vitamin and supplement industry, there's no such thing as an immune-boosting pill, powder, bar, shake, juice, herb, spice, elixir, potion, or food. The best immune boosters are the habits we keep to support the body's innate defenses: a nutritious, diverse diet; regular exercise; restful sleep; and managed stress.

NURTURE YOUR MICROBIOME

A lot has been written about the human microbiome, and it's all the more relevant now in the world of COVID. The microbiome is the link — the biological hinge, if you will — that connects your interactions with your environment (and potential infectious agents) to your immune system.[10] The term *microbiome* comes from the combination of *micro,* for supersmall or microscopic, and *biome,* which refers to a naturally occurring community of life forms occupying a large habitat — in this case, the human body. When I began to study immunology and microbiology as a medical student, the term *microbiome* was not yet on my exams, at least not in the way we talk about it today. Although Joshua Lederberg, a Nobel laureate and microbiologist, is sometimes credited with having coined the term *microbiome* in 2001, the underlying concept and importance of microbiome work hearken back to the beginning of microbial ecology and to Sergei Winogradsky in the 1800s. Lederberg's forte was understanding microbial genetics, and he'd be dazzled by how far we've come since his death in 2008. Roughly 95 percent of the published microbiome scholarship has come in just the past decade, and two-thirds of it only in the past five years.

Today, decoding our microbiome — from the communities deep inside our guts to the colonies that cover our skin — is one of the most promising fields of scientific study. We are at the very beginning of an exciting journey to understanding and leveraging the power of the human microbiome, and the pandemic gives us all the more reason to study this "superorgan" and unlock its secrets. It may hold the future key to our health and ability to combat future pathogens, including COVID's cousins yet to be born.

The ecosystem, or "rainforest," that comprises a human biome includes a diverse collection of microorganisms, mainly bacteria, fungi, yeasts, parasites, and viruses. Their collective genetic material far outnumbers our own DNA. The bacteria that thrive in our intestines are especially important. They have a commanding say in everything about us, from the efficiency and speed of our metabolism to our risk for all manner of ills, COVID-related conditions among them. They assist with digestion and the absorption of nutrients; you can't nourish yourself effectively without them. They also make and release important enzymes and other substances that your body requires but cannot make sufficiently on its own. These include vitamins (notably B vitamins) and neurotransmitters, such as dopamine and serotonin.

An estimated 90 percent of the feel-good hormone serotonin in your body is not made in your brain. It's produced in your digestive tract, thanks to your gut bugs. This intestinal flora and their effects on your hormonal system help you handle stress and even get a good night's sleep.

That's my brief summary on gut bacteria. The main point I want to get across is the following: Of all the actions that these microscopic organisms perform to keep you healthy, perhaps the most vital are the ones that regulate and support your immune system, which is directly tied to your risk for a poor outcome from an infection like COVID. Put simply, your microbial friends help shape your immunity.

The majority — at least 80 percent — of our body's total immune system is made up of gut-associated lymphoid tissue (GALT), the largest mass of lymphoid tissue in the body that's rich in immune cells such as those B and T cells. The GALT lies throughout the intestine, covering a stunningly vast area (up to 300 square meters, which is a little larger than a tennis court!).[11] Indeed, our immune system is headquartered in the gut because the intestinal wall is a biological gateway to the outside world. Aside from skin, it's where we have the greatest chance of encountering foreign material and organisms. The GALT is in constant communication with other immune system cells throughout the body, notifying them if cells in the gut encounter a potentially harmful substance. Because gut bacteria can control certain immune cells and help manage the body's inflammatory pathways, the gut and its inhabitants are said to be your immune system's largest "organ." You may already know that the skin is the largest physical organ. Biologically speaking, the gut and the skin are one and the same, as they present barriers between our insides and outsides that are colonized with microbes. Those microbes can help and hinder how our insides and outsides perform; in fact, the skin and intestinal lining share similar origins in utero during embryonic development. The immune system is dynamic and constantly changes alongside the microbiome throughout our lifetime.

The concept of "you are what you eat" was born when French author Anthelme Brillat-Savarin wrote: "Tell me what you eat and I will tell you what you are," in his 1826 work, *The Physiology of Taste: Or, Meditations on Transcendental Gastronomy.* And now we have plenty of science to show us how this is so, with the microbiome taking center stage. The composition and strength of your microbiome reflect your nutrition and, in turn, your entire physiology. If there's one thing we scientists have learned in just the past decade or so, it's that changes in diet result in adjustments to our microbiome — sometimes in as little as a few days with nutritional tweaks. As our ancestors' diet evolved over time, their gut inhabitants did too, from microbes that could easily break down the fibrous foods plentiful in the early human diet to other microbes better equipped to process the animal proteins, sugars, and starches prevalent after the advent of agriculture and animal husbandry about ten thousand years ago. But as we all know, Westerners have taken the consumption of animal protein, sugars, and starches to the extreme, and the result is a diet high in empty calories and deficient in such nutrients as fiber, essential fatty acids, and other micronutrients that help nourish a healthy microbiome and, in turn, a strong immune system. As the saying goes, we are overfed and undernourished. That is true, but you now understand that your immune system can also be compromised by your diet. If we make bad food choices, we are at greater risk of becoming infected and less able to defend ourselves against a pathogen once it does take hold.

Your gut's microbiome is in constant conversation with the brain through what's called the gut-brain axis. Gut bacteria make chemicals that communicate with the brain through nerves and hormones; the communication is a unique and complex two-way highway. So not only is the gut's community a key to immunity and levels of inflammation, but it's also a linchpin to our entire nervous system. You probably don't think of your gut and brain being strongly connected the way you see your limbs linked up to your brain. But you've no doubt experienced this hidden connection through nerve-racking experiences that leave you, for example, feeling sick to your stomach ("butterflies in your stomach"). The vagus nerve (derived from the Latin word for "wandering" — *vagary* — because this nerve has the longest course of all cranial nerves) is the primary channel of information between the hundreds of millions of nerve cells in your central nervous system and your intestinal nervous system. There's also an axis to your skin to complete the loop, called the gut-brain-skin axis. Hence, when you experience strong emotions, such as fear or embarrassment, your stomach may hurt and your skin may turn "white as a ghost" or flush red.

The vagus nerve is meant to relay messages, but it also helps the health of the gut lining. The gastrointestinal tract is lined with one single layer of surface (epithelial) cells all the way from the esophagus to the anus. The intestinal lining, the body's largest mucosal surface, has three main jobs. First, it serves as the means for the body to obtain nutrients from foods. Second, it blocks the entrance into the bloodstream of potentially harmful particles, chemicals, bacteria, and other organisms and components of organisms that can pose a threat to health. The third function of this cellular barrier is perhaps less well known and deals with its immune function: It contains chemicals called immunoglobulins that bind to bacteria and foreign proteins to prevent them from attaching to the gut's lining. Immunoglobulins are antibodies secreted from immune system cells on the other side of the gut lining and transported into the gut via the intestinal wall. This function ultimately allows such pathogenic organisms and proteins to be pulled from the body, pass on through the intestines, and be excreted.

A key point to remember is that intestinal microbes help control your gut's permeability, or how easily substances pass through the one-cell-thick intestinal epithelium. In addition to the single-cell-thick lining, there are also goblet cells that produce mucus that attaches to the cell wall and makes it "thicker." This process of mucus production depends on back-and-forth interplay with the gut microbiome (the mucus layer typically consists of two layers — and the inner layer is renewed every hour). In other words, your gut's microbiota play a key role in shaping that intestinal barrier structure and its permeability. Microbial imbalances can cause damage to that wall. If there are problems with the integrity of the cells that line the gut due to a microbial disturbance, there can be problems with controlling the passage of nutrients from the digestive tube into the body. And if that gateway is compromised in any way, so is the body's immune system and its resistance to a pathogen like COVID.

The strength and function of your microbiome may play a much bigger role in your immunity and reaction to an infection like COVID than you can imagine — and that science is just beginning to be uncovered. Studies in the past year alone have highlighted the significance of the microbiome in people's prognosis with COVID.[12] Associations found between gut microbiota composition (that is, strains and volume of species) and levels of inflammatory markers in patients with COVID suggest that the gut microbiome is involved in determining the magnitude of the infection. What has been of particular interest to me is the growing possibility that imbalances in the gut's biome, or gut dysbiosis, after COVID clears the body could be a major cause of long-hauler or post-COVID symptoms — brain fog, fatigue, and other persistent symptoms. Experts have also hypothesized that it is an imbalanced gut microbiome that may at least partly explain why older adults and adults with conditions such as obesity or type 2 diabetes seem to be at greater risk of serious COVID illness.

The close relationship between our gut bugs and immunity is likely a two-way street: as infections alter our microbiome, our microbiome alters our immune function and vice versa. Given that the gut is the largest immunological organ in the body and its resident microbes are known to influence immune responses, scientists are focused on teasing out how the gut microbiome affects the immune system's specific response to a COVID infection. And if a connection between the gut microbiota and COVID severity is found, interventions like probiotics or even fecal transplants, to reestablish an individual's healthy microbiome, may help patients in the future. The fecal transplant is an emerging procedure in medicine where a doctor restores the balance of bacteria in a person's gut by taking specially filtered stool from a healthy donor and transferring it into the gastrointestinal tract of the individual with an unhealthy or imbalanced microbiome. Although the procedure is usually reserved for serious gastrointestinal infections such as *C. diff,* future research will surely find other beneficial uses for it in medicine.

The probiotic market, however, has exploded in the past decade. The term *probiotic* is derived from the Latin *pro,* meaning "for," and the Greek word *bios,* meaning "life." Probiotics are the beneficial bacteria you can consume via pill or through such fermented foods as cultured yogurt, cheese, kimchi, and kombucha. Lactic acid fermentation, in fact, is the process by which foods become probiotic, or rich in beneficial bacteria. In this process, good bacteria convert the sugar molecules in the food into lactic acid. In doing so, the bacteria multiply and proliferate. This lactic acid in turn protects the fermented food from being invaded by pathogenic bacteria, because it creates an acidic environment that kills harmful bacteria. That is why lactic acid fermentation is also used to preserve foods. To make fermented foods today, certain strains of good bacteria, such as *Lactobacillus acidophilus,* are introduced to sugar-containing foods to kick-start the process. Yogurt, for instance, is easily made by using a starter culture (strains of live active bacteria) and milk. None of this is new; throughout history, fermented foods have provided probiotic bacteria in the diet.

The ideal composition and species of microbes that make up a healthy microbiome remain unknown, and studies on the value of taking supplemental probiotics have been mixed. We are still in the "we don't know yet" phase as we conduct studies to inform how to support the health of our microbiome. Given how rapidly we are learning about the relationship between gut health and immune health, we may soon be at the point where we will be able to "prescribe" certain strains of probiotics to help treat or even cure a slew of conditions. In fact, certain strains have already been identified that can significantly and positively support the immune system, such as strains in the Bifidobacterium, Lactobacillus, and Saccharomyces genera that are readily available in commercial products, notably fermented foods.

To fully appreciate the microbiome, experts have emphasized to me that it helps to not be reductionist, describing strains as good or bad. After all, studies around the world show that people of different cultures and environments exhibit wildly different microbiomes, which means that one helpful strain of bacteria in one part of the world might be less helpful in another. What seems to be most important is a significant diversity of microbes: the more diverse, the healthier. And there's no better way to consume a rich array of healthy bacteria than to consume them through wholly natural sources, such as sauerkraut, pickles, kimchi, and other fermented vegetables. Once in the gut, these bacteria need to be nurtured by basic lifestyle habits in addition to a good diet, such as regular exercise and restful sleep, which also contribute to the well-being of the microbiome.

Prebiotics are increasingly talked about as well. These are the compounds in certain foods that also promote the growth and activity of beneficial microbes in the gut but are not in and of themselves microbes. They are types of dietary fiber found in many fruits and vegetables, such as chicory root, Jerusalem artichoke, garlic, onion, leek, banana, asparagus, and dandelion greens (toss some of those in a salad!). We live in symbiosis with the microbes in our guts, so it's important to give them a wide variety of things like fibrous fruits and vegetables so they can stay healthy.

MOVE, SLEEP, AND CHILL

Three other keys to maintaining optimal health and immune function are staying active, sleeping well, and reducing stress.

Movement Mitigates COVID

Just twenty-two minutes of moderate exercise a day can strengthen your immune system, and we know now that regular physical activity lessens the severity of COVID — so much so that inactivity is listed by the CDC as a risk factor for severe COVID.[13] For someone who doesn't exercise on a regular basis, 22 minutes a day (150 minutes a week) might sound a bit overwhelming, but those minutes don't have to entail signing up for a gym membership,

355

investing in a treadmill, or revamping your schedule. With the right strategies, you can accomplish your daily exercise goal with very little disruption to your day. Moderate exercise can include walking (at least 4.0 miles an hour), lawn-mowing, and some household chores like vacuuming and mopping.

We humans evolved to move, and move frequently. I know I'm not the first person to tell you this, but it bears repeating that when you avoid routine exercise that gets your heart beating at a faster clip, your blood pumping at a speedier pace, and your skin to sweat, you put yourself at higher risk for the same things a Western diet will do: more inflammation and more chronic disease. Exercise is nature's panacea for the body, providing more health benefits than any drug — and with almost no side effects. It reduces risk for all manner of ills, rapidly flushes out stress hormones, and boosts mood while balancing blood sugar and metabolism in general. Activity improves the health of every organ system, including the brain (and, yes, that all-important lung capacity). If I told you that more than anything else you can do, a mere two minutes of activity every hour can boost your health and make you smarter, wouldn't you want to rethink your sedentary ways? A few years ago, it just hit me one day: we were thinking about it backward. It's not that activity should be thought of as the cure but rather inactivity as the disease. Just move. Every time you are about to sit, ask yourself: Could I stay standing instead? Other tips:

- *Take regular walks.* Walking is so accessible to most people that it's easy to dismiss its benefits. But a brisk walk is one of the most underrated, health-boosting exercises available to humankind. You probably already walk at least a little bit each day. Would it be possible for you to add in a five- or ten-minute walk around the neighborhood before getting in your car to go somewhere? Pair the walk with talking on the phone with a friend or family member or listening to your favorite podcast.

- *Practice short bursts of activity.* Break up your twenty-two-minute minimum with a quick interval training session consisting of four rounds of five exercises for one minute each. These could include body-weight exercises like push-ups, squats, lunges, hip bridges, and jumping jacks. Add in a couple minutes of warm-up and cool-down, and you'll easily hit your twenty-two-minute mark.

- *Pick up an old sport you used to play like tennis or cycling.* If you have kids, play fun games with them that get your heart pumping.
- *Track your movement.* Most smartphones now come with apps that track your miles. Unless you made a serious effort to exercise during the height of stay-at-home orders, many of us fell far behind the 10,000-steps-a-day rule. Accountability goes a long way toward helping us stay on track with fitness goals. A recent study published in the *British Journal of Sports Medicine* found that people walk almost an extra mile per day when using an activity tracker on their phone or watch.[14] And study participants who had fitness trackers with exercise prompts did even more. It doesn't matter how you track your fitness — whether you use smart technology or simply keep a journal, the act of recording your progress will help keep you on track.

People who recover from COVID could

be managing damaged lungs for months that prevent them from engaging in vigorous exercise. Their cardiovascular health could also be compromised as a result of both the effects from the infection and the recovery process that disrupts their fitness routines. Be patient with yourself. In addition to following advice from your doctor, I want to share something that has significantly helped many patients support recovery and strengthen their lungs: performing deep breathing exercises, which also have the added benefit of lessening feelings of anxiety and stress.

Deep breathing can be done anywhere, anytime. A practice twice daily will get you started and give you a foundation. All you have to do is sit comfortably in a chair or on the floor, close your eyes, and make sure your body is relaxed — releasing all tension in your neck, arms, legs, and back. Inhale through your nose for as long as you can, feeling your diaphragm and abdomen rise as your stomach moves outward. Take in a little more air when you think you've reached the top of your lungs. Slowly exhale to a count of twenty, pushing every breath of air from your lungs. Continue for at least five rounds of deep breaths. Another variation on the theme is to try the yawn-smile technique. This exercise incorporates motion with deep breathing, which helps increase coordination and build strength in the arms and shoulders. It also opens up the muscles in your chest to expand the diaphragm. And it's simple: Sit upright on the edge of your bed or in a sturdy chair; reach your arms up straight overhead and create a big stretching yawn; then lower your arms down to your sides and finish by smiling for three seconds. Repeat for one minute. You can find online videos of these practices.

Sleep Supports Immunity

Sleep is medicine.[15] A compelling influx of scientific data shows how sleep acts as a natural drug (like exercise) to recalibrate our body, reorganize our mind and memory, and refresh our cells and tissues down to the molecular level. Sleep restores our body at every level from the brain down to the cells in our toes, so it's no surprise that the relationship between sleep and worsening COVID outcomes is coming into clearer focus. Prolonged sleep deprivation has been found to decrease immune function, promote inflammation, raise levels of cortisol (a key stress hormone), and increase risk of chronic disease. We are learning that the number of circulating, policing immune cells actually peaks at night, which says a lot about the defensive power of sleep.

Sleeping well helps balance the hormones that regulate our biology and immune state; it also affects how well we feel and cope with daily stressors, how fast our metabolism runs, how robustly our brain operates and thinks, and even how our microbiome functions. While it's hard to imagine our sleep having an impact on gut bacteria, new science shows a connection: A healthy microbial gut community helps us sleep and sleep better, and a good night's sleep nurtures diverse, sanguine colonies.

Everyone's sleep needs are different. In general, children need more sleep (ten to twelve hours) than adults (seven to nine). Quality, however, beats quantity. You can sleep for nine hours and still feel tired the next day if you haven't banked enough refreshing deep sleep. The key is to have consistent sleep that moves through all the phases at night repeatedly in sync with the body and fosters a healthy sleep-wake cycle and circadian rhythm. If you want to really know how well you're sleeping and whether you're hitting deep sleep enough throughout the night, wearable devices and apps can help you track — quantify and qualify —

your sleep.

Stress Sinks Immunity[16]

We all experience stress; it's part of life, and it can even be healthy and motivating in many ways. It's the toxic version that we need to minimize because the effects range from nuisances like headaches and bellyaches to problems in mental health like crippling anxiety and depression. Toxic stress is the kind that's unrelenting, prolonged, and so psychologically troubling that it begins to affect our mood, biology, and ability to cope. When the stress hormones start pumping with no end in sight, lots of things can reshape the body, including the power of its immune system.

Stress physiology has come a long way in the past several decades. We have known for a long time about the cascade of events that occur in the body when it is under stress. But we are learning about new conditions tied to stress, including the very chronic conditions that exacerbate a COVID illness. For instance, unabated stress can hurt our microbiome. Experimental studies show that the toxic kind can stall digestion in the small intestine, which can lead to an overgrowth of bacteria there, which then compromises that delicate intestinal barrier.

Unfriendly bacteria are then allowed to grow, crowding out the beneficial bugs — leading to dysbiosis and opening the door to a host of negative effects, some of which can result in chronic conditions in vulnerable people, including a prolonged case of COVID. Once again, this goes to show the interconnectivity of all the systems in the human body.

BUILD MENTAL RESILIENCY

It's no surprise that all measurements — objective and anecdotal — have shown a rise in mental health challenges since the pandemic began. One of the early warning signs was the increase in phone calls to hotlines designed for reporting child and domestic abuse. According to the CDC, from August 2020 to February 2021, the percentage of adults with recent symptoms of anxiety and depression increased from 36.4 percent to 41.5 percent. The emotional toll on people has varied, with some people discovering strengths and others discovering the limits of their coping skills. A variety of factors determine how an individual is affected, including one's age and life stage, childhood adverse events, race, gender, genetics, mental health history, exposure to discrimination and personal life circumstances, financial well-being, access to health care, as well as the range of struggles and losses they've suffered throughout the pandemic. Someone working the front lines in health care, for example, has experienced this event differently from, say, an established accountant who can remain safely sequestered in a home office and Zoom with clients.

The good news is that research has revealed that the majority of people who survive acutely stressful periods like wars, natural disasters, and catastrophes recover without long-term psychological issues. We may be more stressed out, depressed, and anxious than ever before, and every expert I've talked to has said that COVID will change society forever, but research on human resilience shows that people recover from pandemics faster than you'd expect. We have plenty of data showing a rapid recovery after the 1918 flu pandemic. Research also shows that the vast majority of us — about 90 percent of Americans — have experienced a traumatic event but only 6.8 percent of people will have posttraumatic stress disorder.[17] And in follow-up studies of those with PTSD, their symptoms diminish dramatically within three months after the trauma, and almost two-thirds of them eventually recover. It's important, and perhaps comforting, to know that trauma does not necessarily or automatically cause long-term mental illness. There can be psychological distress for sure, as well as sadness and anxiety, but these are normal, temporary reactions that for the most part are manageable. They may even play into the power of your mental resilience. We've all gotten this far in the pandemic, which can now help us build our mental bounce-back muscles.

When I wrote *Keep Sharp,* my focus was on the things we can do to build a resilient brain to avoid cognitive decline and dementias. Although I wrote it prepandemic, all of the ideas and strategies in the book — my five pillars of nourish, move, sleep, continually learn, and connect with others — remain relevant. But let me offer more specifics on how this guidance can be applied in this pandemic age.

The most important insight from all the years I spent researching for my book (which, admittedly, could have easily been titled *Keep Resilient*) is just as appropriate for pandemic times: Your brain is an incredibly pliable organ that can improve as you age. It is an extraordinary thing to consider. Although other organs typically decline through normal wear and tear, the brain can remain robust and actually grow new neurons and networks to support you and your endeavors no matter how old you are. I've met plenty of centenarians with weak hearts but hardy brains (and I've operated on brains that look to be on the brink of death but whose owners still think and form memories like a quick-witted youngster). This means the things you do every day can help you build a better, more pandemic-proof brain. The combination of restorative sleep and exercise, for instance, is an antidote to mental decline — matchless medicine we can't get elsewhere. Sleep tidies memory, and physical activity pumps out substances in the brain that act like Miracle-Gro on brain cells, stimulating their growth and ensuring their survival. This allows us to continually learn new skills and explore new hobbies that are stimulating, de-stressing, and rewarding — all good things for staying mentally resilient. With the temporary loss of many activities that nourish our mental health, such as social gatherings, travel and vacations, and working in an office setting with colleagues, we've had to get creative. And that's okay. Here are some additional tips:

Cut your consumption of media calories.
Think about what media sources you're
following and how often you're checking
them. Instead of scrolling through endless headlines or binge-watching another
TV show, call a friend and connect or
go for a walk outside with a loved one.
Nature loves to suck up your worries.
Too much media consumption can make
us feel that we're losing control of our
lives. Research shows that when we shift
our focus to what we can control, we see
meaningful and lasting differences in our
well-being, health, and performance.

Maintain strict structure. Just as the body
loves homeostasis, a stable equilibrium
or balance across its systems, the mind
loves predictability, order, and routines.
This allows you to adapt quickly to
unexpected changes and challenges.
Create daily to-do lists; set goals; organize your spaces including where you
work; stick to a regular schedule for eating, exercising, and sleeping even on
weekends; and commit to an end-of-day
ritual that's calming, such as reading,
taking a warm bath, or walking through
your neighborhood while listening to
your favorite music.

Keep connections thriving. One of the more

devastating epidemics that has surely arisen from the pandemic is loneliness. Since the start of the pandemic, 67 percent of Americans — two in three people — say they feel more alone than ever before, and many admit to crying for the first time in years.[18] This breaks my heart and makes me want to emphasize with more passion than ever how important it is to call, video-chat with, email, or write letters to the people we care about. We need those deep conversations. Social support is proven to strengthen resilience by increasing our sense of control and self-esteem. Sociality also has positive neural outcomes: it actually deactivates circuits in the brain that trigger fear and anxiety. Put another way: When we connect with others, we hot-wire our brain's calming centers while taming its emotional reflexes.

Use apps that help you practice mind-body medicine. From apps that help you meditate, to those that allow you to join online groups to share your experiences and socialize, there's no shortage these days of programs to help you build resilience. Harvard University's Center on the Developing Child maintains a website with links to national and international resources that can help with a variety of concerns related to the pandemic whether you have children or not: https://developingchild.harvard.edu/resources/covid-19-resources/.

Seek professional help. The explosion of telemedicine has made finding a licensed therapist often only a swipe or call away. As my favorite Olympian Michael Phelps says, "You don't have to wait for things to get that bad. Therapy isn't just for people struggling with serious mental illness." He's teamed up with the maker of an app that helps anyone find a qualified therapist easily, conveniently, and affordably because he knows personally that it sometimes takes a team effort to beat depression and anxiety. Pandemic-related stress aside, one in four people around the world experience a mental health issue, and more than half of American adults do not receive treatment. Professional treatment used to be exclusive, but no longer. And it's there for our children as well. According to the CDC, the proportion of mental health–related emergency room visits for children ages twelve to seventeen increased 31 percent in 2020 compared with 2019. The CDC maintains a comprehensive parental resource kit online that is broken down by age group, from early childhood to young adults.

Use food to boost mood. The idea that you are what you eat applies to mental health too. In addition to microbiome research soaring in scientific circles, so is "nutritional psychiatry."[19] This burgeoning new field of medicine looks at the relationship between food and mental wellness with a nod to the microbiome's role in this biological partnership. Good nutrition feeds and supports a healthy microbiome that ultimately has an impact on brain health, including the production of compounds in the body that foster optimal thinking and mental well-being. Scientists have long focused on how food affects our physical health, specifically our metabolism and heart health. But now the attention is turning to food's surprising connection with mental health as a growing body of research points to how daily sustenance plays into our moods and brain biology. As comforting as our sugary, high-fat delights might seem when we're stressed or depressed, large population studies reveal that people who eat a lot of nutrient-dense foods — more fruits and vegetables, nuts and seeds, beans and legumes, fish, eggs, and fermented products like yogurt — experience less anxiety and depression and report greater levels of happiness and overall life satisfaction. The food-mood connection may seem anecdotal, but we finally have well-designed studies to demonstrate the power of food in our moods and mental resiliency.[20] This does not mean a kale salad and sardines can cure mental illness, but what we choose to eat is arguably one of the most underestimated and under-appreciated ingredients to mental health. It won't cost you more to switch to healthier foods either. In one of the recent studies to test the benefits of food on mental health, participants who switched from sugary cereals to oatmeal, pizza to vegetable stir-fries, and sausage to seafood lowered their weekly grocery bills.

Throughout the pandemic, we've been told that "we're all in this together." This slogan is fitting because we must maintain that mentality as we face future threats. And this often means making the pandemic-proof future a family affair.

CHAPTER 8
O: ORGANIZE FAMILY

**LEARN HOW TO LIVE EVERYDAY
LIFE ANEW (WITH A TWIST)**

Will we ever look at a cough or sneeze in the same way again? How do we plan for parents in need of assisted living or a nursing home? How do we get our kids back on track in school? What should we know before taking a big trip? Does it make sense to spend more on health insurance to deal with any long-term effects from COVID?

We are all in this together, and every family would do well to get organized in ways they probably hadn't thought about prepandemic. After speaking to infectious disease experts, social scientists, and many individuals who have suffered through COVID, I've put together a ten-point family checklist that addresses the best strategies for living with COVID, given it may be in our environment indefinitely. We all have to factor in COVID when making decisions now. As we return to a new normal mindfully, we will continue to grapple with uncertainty, the aftermath of the pandemic, COVID's potential to resurge, as well as the possibility of a new maniacal pathogen arising and threatening the world. As I finished this book, I transitioned my *Coronavirus: Fact vs. Fiction* podcast to a new one, called *Chasing Life*. We're all ready to imagine the next chapter of our lives and find a balance between self-care and productivity. It's time to chase life again. And we have to start somewhere. Follow these ten COVID-friendly commandments to put you and yours in the best position to pandemic proof:

Keep Up with Checkups, Cancer Screenings, and Booster Shots

As the entire world faced off against an insidious globe-trotting virus, our focus temporarily drifted away from the chronic, noncommunicable health issues such as heart disease, cancer, diabetes, and dementia, which continue to affect millions of people and cost untold billions of dollars a year to treat. We must get back to our regular checkups and annual tests to treat and prevent these issues. And, yes, we are all anxious to put COVID in the rearview mirror, but we must not forget COVID's potential to crop up again and again. Staying up to date with booster shots will be key to maintaining community immunity and preventing another pandemic.

Doctors and hospitals have learned how to protect patients from potential COVID exposures, so you no longer have to worry about deciding when and if to receive care or have elective surgery. If there's a local outbreak, doctors and hospitals will snap alert, and you will simply have to follow their lead and abide by their safety measures.

Fill the Thriving Gap
The pandemic caused widespread slowdowns in our children's educational trajectories while also amplifying gaps across racial and socioeconomic lines. This was most pronounced among students from disadvantaged homes, where access to remote learning with reliable Internet was difficult, if not impossible, or kids struggled with online platforms and lack of adequate parental supervision. It's hard to be on Zoom all day long, learning and interacting, no matter how old you are. While it's tempting to call it "learning loss," that's not the best term. Our kids may not have lost as

much as we think and could have actually gained a lot in experiencing this pandemic. They may have lost time in a traditional classroom, but that doesn't mean they lost skills, knowledge, memories, or the capacity for future wisdom. It was Plutarch who wrote, "The mind is not a vessel to be filled but a fire to be kindled." And they are ready for a rekindling.

After speaking to superintendents in school districts all over the country, I am optimistic that we will address many of these gaps with public measures by offering high-dosage tutoring, extending school years, and partnering with community organizations. Make no mistake: None of this is ideal, but educators across the country have emphasized to me that they view the pandemic as an interruption and not a permanent regression in our kids' education. Many school districts have led the charge to get kids back in school safely.

When I wrote and recorded the audio book *Childhood, Interrupted,* I spoke to child psychologists around the country to learn their concerns and their plans so that I could apply those lessons to my own three girls.[1] For starters, they reminded me that the *thriving gap,* a much better term than *learning loss,* doesn't include just the academic element. It's also the social and emotional gap, especially for teenagers, who'd rather be with their friends than anywhere else. Especially as kids are increasingly vaccinated, make sure those social connections are nurtured once again.

"For both older and younger kids, they are remarkably resilient," said scientist and psychologist Angela Duckworth who founded the nonprofit Character Lab to collect science-backed data to help kids thrive.[2] "Sometimes people think that resilience is the exception — but it's actually the rule." According to Duckworth, it helps to frame the pandemic from a perspective that doesn't dwell on the loss and brokenness, and instead, ask, *What can I learn?* and *What can I do going forward?* That small mental shift in a parent's mind will shape how a child reacts and chooses to think about things. For example, literacy is the foundation to learning, and practicing literacy with your child is something every parent can do at home. Kids learn every day, whether they are in a traditional academic environment or on their computers in their rooms with classmates online, starting to ride a bike in the neighborhood, or playing video games with friends through the Internet. Learning is not binary; it's complicated. Our kids will learn new skills they should have learned last year. Maybe that's a good thing, because in years to come, we'll likely find that our children are not only "caught up" with their learning but they've surpassed it because the pandemic bestowed on them an experience that teaches like nothing else can.

Choose Health Care Plans Wisely

Medical debt spiked $2.8 billion, or about 6.5 percent, from the end of May 2020 to the end of March 2021, and past-due medical debt grew by nearly 9 percent, from $19.6 million to $21.4 million.[3] People who got really sick without proper health coverage or who faced ongoing health problems and endless doctor visits to treat long-haul COVID suffered huge economic fallouts. Many people lost health care coverage altogether with their jobs.

The Affordable Care Act (ACA) has been a solution for many people who would otherwise not have access to medical insurance (when it's open enrollment, you can buy plans on HealthCare.gov — some without any premium if you qualify). The ACA bars insurers from discriminating against people with medical conditions or charging them more than healthier policyholders. This is especially good news for former COVID patients who could face a range of long-term physical or mental effects, including lung damage, heart problems, or neurological conditions including depression. Although some of these issues will heal with time, others may turn out to be long-standing problems. When shopping for health insurance, here are a few important tips:

- *Make sure you choose an ACA-qualified plan,* and shop around to consider all the plans available to you in your region. Non-ACA plans may be enticing for their lower price tag, but they offer less comprehensive coverage and are not eligible for federal subsidies that help people who qualify pay for the cost of the premiums. A short-term, limited-duration plan is never going to be the right decision. Spend some time doing your homework, and ask lots of questions.
- *Stay in your network.* Make sure the doctors, specialists, and hospitals you use are in your plan's network. If you find yourself seeking out-of-network care, you will pile on debt because those bills will come in and you won't have coverage. Sometimes working

with a broker for health care policies can help you navigate this more easily (brokers don't typically charge you for their services since they get paid by insurance companies). If you're a COVID survivor, factor in the possibility of needing more coverage for more doctor visits and access to specialists. As I'll note later, you'll want access to multidisciplinary clinics where teams of doctors from various fields of medicine work together. HealthCare.gov has a "find local help" button that can refer you by zip code to navigators, assisters, and brokers. When you're looking for coverage to meet each individual family member's specific needs, it helps to speak to someone about what's available and within your budget.

- *Factor in deductibles.* You must meet a deductible before the better part of financial assistance kicks in. In most cases, the higher the premium you pay, the lower the deductible will be. But getting past a high deductible can be difficult if you've chosen a plan with a low premium and you need complex care at once or expensive prescription drugs. Those with ongoing health conditions need to carefully weigh the expected annual out-of-pocket costs for various health plans. And be wary of "zero-deductible" plans, because these may have hidden costs you don't realize until you're billed. Read all the fine print.

Rebuild Emergency Funds and Financial Cushions

For many families, the pandemic led to financial distress as people lost jobs and had medical bills piling up. Any emergency funds, if they existed, have been drained. Now is the time to create a post-COVID spending plan that prioritizes establishing (or reestablishing) that emergency fund — before paying off debt or planning lavish vacations (I know; after all this isolation, the urge to "get back" to life might lead to overspending on all the things that we have missed most). According to disaster financial planners I interviewed, you should aim to save up to a full year's worth of living expenses in your family emergency fund. Prioritize bills you must pay (e.g., rent, mortgage, car, insurance), and funnel as much cash as you can toward your emergency fund until it's full. The goal is to remain as flexible as possible with cash to best prepare for another pandemic.

Personal finance expert Suze Orman maintains a lot of practical advice and tools on her site, SuzeOrman.com. Although she doesn't usually advise that people prioritize saving over paying off high-interest debt, she also knows these aren't typical times. During the acute phase of a pandemic, saving cash above all else is sometimes the right strategy as long as you have mapped out a plan to eventually pay attention to debt and credit scores later. However, no matter which phase we're in, a priority to save and maintain those emergency funds is always good advice. In Orman's words, "An emergency savings fund is not an investment. It is security. It is peace of mind. It is protection." To that I'll add, it's smart pandemic preparation.

Have an Advance Health Directive in Place
It took many families a grim trip to the hospital with severe COVID to realize they had never thought about end-of-life decisions. Many families faced abrupt decisions about the kind of care they wanted for themselves or their loved ones. And many of these difficult conversations had to happen over the phone since the pandemic

prevented families from entering hospitals to help loved ones fight through the illness by the bedside or, worse, prepare to die. When the pandemic struck, people filled out advance directives at five times the rate they had before. Unfortunately, fewer than a third of healthy US adults have an advance directive. This legal document can give instructions about the kind of medical care you prefer if you become seriously ill and are at the end of your life. You can specify the types of medical treatments you do and do not wish to receive and can designate someone who will make sure that your health care decisions are followed. Would you want everything possible done to keep your vital organs working? If your kidneys start to fail, would you want to be put on dialysis? What if you need chest compressions, placement of a breathing tube, or defibrillation?

You do not want your family to be making these kinds of decisions while in crisis mode. Advance medical directives are often included in traditional will and trust packages, but they can be executed on their own. (As a resource, AARP offers links to free, downloadable advance directive forms for each state. For some states, living will and health care proxy forms are combined into one document. For other states, the forms are separate. Another resource to check out is the University of Pennsylvania's free tool at OurCare Wishes.org.)

I recommend every family make it a goal to organize these important legal documents no matter how much value they think is in their "estate." A family or estate attorney can help draft and execute these important documents, including durable power of attorney (designating who can make financial and other decisions when someone is no longer able) and instructions for where assets go once you're gone — even if those assets are purely sentimental, like your collection of sports memorabilia. These documents tend to be lengthy and detailed, and they specify some of the most practical but difficult decisions that you must eventually face. Forgoing these documents can be financially ruinous to families — triggering unexpected medical bills left to loved ones dealing with the financial aftermath. When a person does not have an advance directive, extraordinary and aggressive measures to save a life could be taken with enormous costs. I realize that these conversations are not fun to have and involve tough, serious hypotheticals to consider, but ask anyone who has been through the experience of *not* having these documents in place when they were needed, and he or she will strongly encourage you to get them done. Look at completing an advance directive as a belated holiday gift to your family this season.

Travel Smartly

This one is easy: Follow the CDC's guidelines to know where it's relatively safe to travel both domestically and internationally (surprise: Domestic travel is not inherently safer than international travel if there are hot spots at home and COVID-free places abroad). Even if you're vaccinated, you'll want to plan ahead and do your homework. Before booking lodging or transportation, find out the company's COVID cleaning procedure, whether there's a vaccination and face mask policy, and what happens if you decide to cancel. Check for restrictions at your destination and anywhere you might stop along the way. Don't know whether to brave flying or go by car? Both bear risks. Most viruses don't spread easily on flights because of how air is exchanged and filtered in airplanes. But crowded flights, security lines, and airport terminals make physical distancing difficult. Once at your destination, follow local rules and recommendations, and you'll stay safe. Consider buying what's called Cancel for Any Reason travel insurance (standard travel insurance likely won't cover COVID-related trip changes), which will generally reimburse you 75 percent of your travel costs.

Here are some additional tips:

- Aim for vacations that keep you mostly outdoors where spread of the virus is minimal.
- Look for all-in-one resorts that offer an abundance of space, and maintain strict COVID-sensitive protocols. Or rent a house where exposure risk is low in the area and the rental company has implemented exhaustive cleaning protocols and checklists. No matter where you are, your biggest risk of infection remains prolonged indoor, face-to-face contact with unmasked people. One of the most important factors to consider when renting is who you're going to share your space with.
- Take a guided trip with a respected operator that organizes a COVID-safe journey. If you want to go on a cruise, you might want to save long-distance Caribbean or European voyages for the post-pandemic era, and instead, stay within the United States by selecting

one of many small ships that travel our finest water routes, such as the Great Lakes, Chesapeake Bay, and the Mississippi, Snake, and Columbia Rivers. Coastal communities on the Atlantic, Pacific, or Gulf offer trips on their nearby waters. Because cruise liners may not mandate vaccination for passengers or crew, it's up to you to ask questions and choose the liners that have the safest, strictest COVID protocols. The nature of a cruise ship — tight quarters, shared spaces, lots of contact with strangers — makes these voyages uniquely risky when there's a bug on board. Remember, it only took one confirmed individual to infect hundreds on the *Diamond Princess* in 2020.

Vaccine passports may be necessary while traveling. This can entail physical cards or cell phone apps that show your vaccinated status. There probably won't be a universal system, so you'll have to comply with whatever passport rules are established. In the United States, it's up to individual states, universities, and businesses to decide whether they want to require such passports. At this writing, there are no plans for a universal federal vaccination database or a mandate. If you're carrying around your CDC-issued vaccination card in your wallet, make a digital copy and save the original in a safe, locked place at home or in a bank safety deposit box where you keep other important documents. Until vaccines are approved for all children, traveling with unvaccinated kids adds another complicated layer. You'll want to continue to protect them as much as possible from exposure, which means continuing to wear masks, wash hands, and physical distance from other people. While zero risk is not a practical goal, we should still do the basics to minimize risk as much as possible without sacrificing a fulfilling life.

Rethink Long-Term Care Facilities for Aging Parents

Some of the most heartbreaking images from the early days of the pandemic were taken in nursing homes and retirement communities ravaged by the virus. Many assisted-living facilities became death traps for older people who were exposed to the virus. The combination of age and underlying health conditions in a closed, shared setting made them exceptionally vulnerable: About 8 percent of people who live in US long-term care facilities have died of COVID — nearly 1 in 12.[4] In nursing homes, the figure is nearly 1 in 10. Throughout the pandemic, long-term care facility deaths made up over a third of all US deaths.

Although these places should now have a plan to protect residents, workers, volunteers, and visitors from a COVID outbreak, I believe most people will think carefully about sending a beloved family member to one of these facilities. Many factors make these spaces vulnerable to viral and bacterial diseases: frequent physical contact between residents and staff, employees who shuffle in and out and work in many facilities, and residents sharing rooms where physical distancing is difficult.

Problems with infection control in these settings predate the pandemic. A May 2020 report from the US Government Accountability Office found that four in five nursing homes surveyed between 2013 and 2017 were cited for deficiencies in infection prevention and control, leading the Centers for Medicare and Medicaid Services (CMS) to announce tougher rules for infection-control inspections and enforcement.[5] The CMS now requires nursing homes to tell residents and their families or representatives within twelve hours if a COVID case is confirmed on-site. The information must also be reported to the CDC and is compiled in an online data set where you can find week-by-week case numbers at individual facilities.

Although we now can rely on vaccines to keep residents and staff safer, we cannot assume that everyone's vaccination status will remain the same. Long-term care facilities have been one of the great success stories of vaccination for COVID, as rates of the disease in nursing homes decreased by more than 80 percent since vaccination began, but nearly a quarter of nursing home and assisted care facility staff have no plans to get the vaccine. Many more may skip booster shots in the future. Note that unlike nursing homes, assisted-living facilities do not typically have federal oversight. For example, the CMS rules on disclosing COVID cases to residents and family members do not apply to assisted-living facilities, which are licensed by the states.

Choose nursing homes and assisted-living facilities carefully. If you have a loved one in an assisted-living community and have questions or concerns about its COVID caseload and protocols, contact the facility and ask to speak to an administrator. You can also raise issues to your state's department of health or department of aging. Consider these questions to ask at a potential long-term care facility:

- What are your protocols for testing residents and staff?
- Do you mandate vaccines? (I would choose a transparent facility where vaccination for COVID is a condition of employment. In fact, vaccination rates for staff should be made readily available to interested family members. Note that in institutions where influenza vaccination is mandatory, vaccine rates of around 98 percent can be achieved compared to vaccination rates below 50 percent in health care facilities where it's not mandatory.)
- What happens when there is an outbreak?
- What safety protocols are in place to prevent a COVID outbreak?
- How do you maintain and support your staff? (Retaining excellent workers is key to a good facility.)

Be Okay with Shifting Social Circles
Pandemics are divisive by nature as people wrestle with how to respond. COVID has

been no different, as experienced by families and friends who spar over public health measures and the severity of the pandemic. Everyone has his or her own version of what's right. I think we all know someone who didn't abide by the rules at the height of the outbreak and tested our tolerance for such behavior. The politicization of the pandemic in the United States has made it especially hard to maintain social graces with so many competing values. We've all had to modify our social norms in ways that complicate how we work, interact with others, and generally go about our days. When our lives are at risk, other people's opinions over what it means to be safe suddenly bear more weight than casual differences on matters unrelated to health and wellness. Things can get tricky when people's boundaries and perceived levels of safety are in conflict.

Relationships may be permanently affected by this pandemic, and that's okay. Many people's social lives were already fraying before the pandemic, and the winnowing to essential, first-tier people may have been a relief. There's solace in a pared-down social life. We had a chance to reset our social lives and set new boundaries. The pandemic revealed which relationships are worth keeping and nourishing (and, yes, friendship breaks are entirely normal regardless of a pandemic).

With life returning to a semblance of normalcy, how do you respond to people who make you feel uncomfortable by inviting you to attend their big indoor party where you believe that many guests are unvaccinated? Be honest, and kindly tell them you don't feel comfortable spending time with them in a particular setting. Think about your relationship — what you know about the people, where they are coming from — and determine how to interact with them. This isn't about trying to change their minds. It's about standing up for your own needs, feelings, and values. On my podcast, I spent a lot of time speaking to scientists about the virus, but also about how they navigate their own lives, given their background. A few themes emerged.

Use "I" statements so you don't come across as accusatory: "I am not comfortable." And if they tease you or get angry, say, "I hear you. I might feel the same way if I were in your position." You can go further: "I'm just not willing or able to do this. This is about me. I'm now feeling like I'm not being heard, and that's really hard, given our friendship. Can we talk about that?" In some instances, you may have to walk away from a conversation and stop engaging. Avoid jumping into heated, overly charged conversations where there's a lack of empathy and compassion. If you're tempted to tell someone, "You're crazy!" it's not going to go well. And if you feel the need to challenge someone's thoughts or ideas about pandemic behavior, start with, "Where are you hearing that?" or "Please tell me more about your perspective so I can try to understand." Listen to their concerns without judgment. You want to address their anxiety with compassion and show you care about their welfare. This helps build trust. It also validates their concerns. You can even share your own doubts and worries and point to resources that helped you make a particular decision. Present information you can back up with an apolitical article or post from a credible source to which the person might respond positively. Try and give them a sense of ownership of the new knowledge. Keep the conversation collaborative rather than one-sided, like you're both learning and taking things as they come step by step.

It's important to continue to build connections with other people for your emotional well-being and general health, but not with people who make you feel unsafe.

Research has shown that pointing fingers, blaming, or shaming anyone for their behaviors (or lack thereof in the case of vaccine refusal) is not helpful. Remember: *Share; don't shame* is my motto. If your friends are hesitant to get vaccinated, share your great experience about how freeing it is to be so protected from COVID. The majority of people who are hesitant to get vaccinated are not stupid or selfish. They simply want more information and reassurances from people they trust — their friends, mentors, doctors, colleagues, and family members. That means you and me.

Find a New Work-Life Balance

I think I speak for millions of people when I say never has my work-life balance been more disrupted than during this pandemic. We got sent to our rooms for over a year. We actually began to miss long commutes that allowed us some peace and quiet and time to reflect (I missed long flights to destinations for reporting). The pandemic blurred the lines — and passage of time — between work and play. One woman put it perfectly: "I feel less like I'm working from home and more like I'm living at work." I won't even mention what it's been like for people raising kids. But work and life should not compete, and it helps to think of work as merely part of life, and we get to choose how it appears. With many people returning to traditional offices full- or part-time in a hybrid model, it's key to strike a new balance. Some tips:

- *Make a mental commitment to boundaries.* Have a designated workspace and time, choosing your work hours (if possible) to take place when you're most creative and productive. Do not respond immediately to messages outside those working hours. For me, this means organizing my day like a surgeon — being precise, methodical, and procedural. If your office uses chat apps or Slack, change your status to "off work" or "do not disturb" when you're done with working hours. Be willing to say, "I have a commitment this evening but can look at that tomorrow." As a boss once said to me, "*No* can be a full sentence in these situations." You don't have to have plans to want some time for yourself outside work. Communicate transparently with your colleagues about your work hours and schedule. We can be more flexible with where we work, and that's a good thing. If you find yourself anxious and socially awkward as you ease back into old work settings, be patient with yourself. A little social anxiety after more than a year spent mostly at a safe distance from others is totally normal.

- *Set realistic expectations* on a daily and weekly basis for yourself at work and at home, even if they occur in the same place.
- *Establish a nonnegotiable twenty-minute transition period in between work and play* during which you maintain a ritual (e.g., meditating, reading, journaling, walking around the block) that calms and invigorates you.
- *Reset the division of labor.* When the late Supreme Court justice's son misbehaved, school officials often called Ruth Bader Ginsberg. She reminded the school that her son had two parents and asked it to alternate between them. Clearly, that was several decades ago, but the lesson remains just as relevant today. Women have suffered disproportionately during the pandemic, with many leaving the workforce entirely or downshifting careers. Couples need to work as a team and

accept that some days will be better than others.

Learn to Live with Germs

We cringe when we touch a dirty ATM keypad on the street or accidentally inhale someone's sneeze nearby. Nothing looks the same anymore. Even a public restroom feels like a hazard zone (indeed, as MIT researchers have shown, "toilet plume," an airborne dispersal of microscopic particles created by the flush of a toilet, is a real phenomenon and, in some cases, a valid public health concern).[6] It's not easy to transmit many pathogenic germs, including COVID, on surfaces, but our perceptions of what's dirty or germy have definitely changed. Between the copious bottles of hand sanitizer, disinfecting sprays, and antimicrobial products, you'd think we're cleansing the world and sterilizing ourselves. But we are awash in microbes whether we like it or not, and as you have now learned, many of our microbial comrades are beneficial to human health. My brief description of the human microbiome is one example of how friendly germs are part of who we are. They can be our best friends. We could never rid ourselves of all germs and should not want to do so. At some point, as COVID infection rates abate with community immunity, we'll need to dial back our antimicrobial efforts lest we harm our immune systems paradoxically by depriving them of their continual education.

It was the British epidemiologist David Strachan who in 1989 used the alliterative term *hygiene hypothesis,* making the case that exposure to infections during childhood provides a good defense against allergies in later life.[7] He proposed that a lower incidence of infection in early childhood could be an explanation for the twentieth-century uptick in allergic diseases and asthma. In the *British Medical Journal* (now just called the *BMJ*), Strachan published his early findings that children in larger households had fewer instances of hay fever because they are exposed to germs by older siblings. This led to further research showing that a lack of early-childhood exposure to microbes can increase an individual's susceptibility to disease. It established the theory that a rising incidence of chronic allergic diseases such as hay fever (allergic rhinitis), eczema, and asthma may be an inevitable price to be paid for freedom from the burden of killer infectious diseases. The hygiene hypothesis, also called the *microbial hypothesis* or *old friends hypothesis* to avoid the overemphasis on cleanliness, has evolved over the past thirty-some years with plenty of critics debating its finer points, but there's scientific consensus that certain exposures promote health and being too clean can backfire. The hypothesis has also been extended to explain conditions as diverse as food allergies, autoimmune diseases (e.g., type 1 diabetes and multiple sclerosis), inflammatory bowel disease, some cancers, and even Alzheimer's disease.[8]

The concept is analogous to what happens when you build muscle mass and strength through weight training. By gradually increasing the weight of objects you lift over time, you teach and prime your muscles to work and more easily lift those heavy things. According to immunologists I interviewed, the same idea is true for the immune system. To fight off an infection, which is a "weight" of sorts, the immune system must train and learn by fighting off contaminants found in everyday life. Systems that aren't exposed to contaminants have trouble with the heavy lifting of fighting off infections. We must still be hygienic during periods such as flu season, but it should not become an obsession. Remember, we need to tap-dance our way through our existence on the planet, not isolate ourselves from it. Once we've reached community immunity with COVID, we should end our hygiene zealotry and start lifting our weights again.

When Dr. B. Brett Finlay, a professor in the department of microbiology and immunology at the University of British Columbia, teaches about the microbiome, he points out that our bodies contain at least as many bacterial cells as human cells and that before the pandemic, only one of the top ten causes of death in America, influenza, was attributable to an infectious disease that someone could "catch."[9] Nearly all the rest, such as heart disease, cancer, brain disease and stroke, diabetes, and obesity, are associated with poor microbiome health or dysfunction. Dr. Finlay's 2021 paper raised the alarm about the microbial fallout that may follow in the pandemic's wake. "You can't change your genes, but you can change your microbes," he says. "They're our friends."

SPECIAL NOTE FOR LONG-HAULERS

Of all the mysterious features of COVID, its long-term effects in some people puzzle even the most brilliant doctors and scientists. For most people, COVID is a disease that involves a few weeks of discomfort, or, for the sick or elderly, it is one that can lead to hospitalization or death. But for others, it's a disease that waxes and wanes over time with no end in sight, even after a relatively mild or asymptomatic case in the initial stage. It becomes an ongoing hardship for both the individual with the illness and the entire family around that person. And it demands an inclusive, collective approach as a family unit to help a loved one through the challenges.

Research suggests that 50 to 80 percent of people who recover from COVID experience at least some lingering aftereffects three months after infection.[10] Although estimates vary, at least 10 percent (and upwards of 30 percent) of people who get COVID could become long-haulers indefinitely whose prognosis is uncertain, which can be scary. In the United States, that amounts to nearly 10 million people left with prolonged symptoms. This condition is so debilitating that it has delayed or derailed careers, kept people from going back to work, and made everyday living and completion of the simplest tasks excruciating.

We need to put our arms around these people and take care of them, learning from their experience so we can formulate the best treatments and cures. Despite the staggering numbers, there are no clear diagnoses, no standard care, and no national guidelines for how these patients should be treated. Once we can better define long-haul COVID, my hope is we can help patients manage and treat their disease like any other chronic condition through the right medicine and healthy lifestyle. The medical community is rapidly creating standardized definitions and guidelines of care. Despite some similarities among long-haulers — often women in their thirties, forties, and fifties — we don't have any diagnostic criteria. Images of the lungs or heart can't help us identify post-COVID illness. That COVID can become chronic partly explains why patients who have had it bear a 60 percent higher risk of death between one and six months after getting sick than those who never had the infection. And patients who have had COVID also show a 20 percent greater chance of needing more medical care and medication over the six months after their diagnosis. Chronic conditions breed other chronic conditions, and the body can become vulnerable to a spectrum of illness and disorder.

Dr. Francis Collins, director of the National Institutes of Health (Dr. Fauci's boss), has announced a major commitment to understanding long-haul COVID with an initiative worth $1.15 billion over four years to fund investigations of the conditions associated with it. And those conditions are extensive, often occurring in waves: extreme fatigue, fevers, muscle aches, heart palpitations and irregular heart rhythms, changes in blood pressure, shortness of breath; headache, confusion, dizziness, loss of hearing, tinnitus, and inability to concentrate ("brain fog"); diarrhea, nausea, vomiting, and loss of taste and smell or phantom smells and tastes; mouth sores, twitchy muscles, eye infections, hair loss, and skin conditions; as well as psychiatric and mood conditions such as anxiety, paranoia, delirium, and depression. Long-haul neurological symptoms like anxiety disorders and depression seem to be distinct from neurological complications found in the acute phase, such as a stroke or seizures. And while we don't know yet if COVID can have very long-term consequences, such as a recovered twentysomething living with an increased risk for dementia or Alzheimer's disease later in life, the current thinking suggests COVID is primarily an inflammatory vascular disease with downstream effects. In other words, while it may not cause brain disease in and of itself, patients may still have similar symptoms.

"I think of COVID as a medical illness with multiple related sequelae that can fast-forward or trigger cognitive decline and brain disease, but so can so many other things," says Dr. Richard Isaacson, a neurologist at New York–Presbyterian/Weill Cornell Medical Center and founder of its Alzheimer's Prevention Clinic. The vast majority of his patients go back to their baseline cognitive status after recovering from COVID. Whether the virus directly attacks the brain remains debated, as studies fail to detect the COVID virus in the brains of people who died of it. But we do know that during the acute phase of infection, there may be inflammation in the brain, an autoimmune reaction, and an impairment of the autonomic nervous system's ability to regulate certain bodily processes. There may also be vascular changes that underlie some of the neurological conditions doctors see in patients. Research scientists are beginning to document two big driving forces in the long-haul phenomenon: organ and blood vessel damage caused by the infection and an immune overreaction, or the virus lingering in the body to perpetuate problems.

This last idea, that COVID can remain

hidden somewhere in the body, would put it in the same bucket as other infections that can lie dormant and strike later on such as chicken pox and shingles. Research has also revealed that COVID may cause changes to an infected person's genes, influencing their behavior. To be clear, the virus is not changing your DNA but it can impact how genes express themselves dynamically, which can impact the inflammatory response in the body. Research scientists at Texas Tech University Health Sciences Center have found that exposure to the infamous COVID spike protein alone was enough to change baseline gene expression in the airway cells of infected patients, suggesting that the first COVID symptoms someone develops may initially result from the spike protein interacting with the cells directly, even more than the infection itself.[11]

In many ways, that brings us back to the beginning of this part of the book and the concept of epigenetics. External forces act on our genetic code every day. These signals have the power to change how our genes behave and how our DNA is turned into messages and building blocks for our body — which means you have the ability to alter, for better or worse, the activity of your DNA. By definition, epigenetics is the study of how your behaviors and environment can cause changes that affect the way your genes work. Unlike genetic changes, epigenetic changes are reversible and do not change your DNA sequence, but they can change how your body reads a DNA sequence.[12] Put another way, epigenetic changes affect gene expression to turn genes "on" and "off." Since your environment and behaviors, such as diet and exercise, can result in epigenetic changes, it is easy to see the connection between your genes and your behaviors and environment. And it's how we get to decide which genetic switches we want to turn on or off.

Now, how does an infection like COVID become an epigenetic force? Although we all know that our environment and our lifestyle choices, such as what we eat and how we exercise, play a significant role in our health, we often don't think about the subtler forms of "environment" that have an impact on us, such as an infection. An individual's response to COVID and whether he or she goes on to develop a long-haul illness are likely the result of a complex interplay of genetic, epigenetic, and environmental factors. I believe we will find patterns in the data from long-haulers and be able to better predict who is more likely to have a prolonged illness.

Long-haul recovery programs are appearing throughout the country and at places like Mount Sinai Hospital in New York where a post-COVID clinic has been established. When Diana Berrent launched Survivor Corps in spring 2020 to help mobilize and collect data and research tools for patients and doctors alike, she didn't expect the following to grow so fast.[13] But it's a testament to the problem and the ever-expanding need for answers and treatments. Berrent was among the first people to contract COVID in New York back in March 2020. She went on to have long-haul symptoms for months after testing negative for the virus, with those symptoms ranging from headaches and stomach issues to glaucoma, increasing her risk for blindness. Her preteen son also contracted the virus and still had symptoms nine months later.

"It's like we've lost limbs that we now must find a way to grow back," one survivor explained to me. That analogy is useful, because there's no such thing as growing back an arm or a leg (if only that were possible!). If your leg has been amputated, your new normal likely involves learning how to walk again with a prosthetic device. It's probably not helpful to yearn for life before the amputation and regret all that you can no longer do. Such obsessive thinking about the past can hinder progress in the recovery. The same goes for COVID survivors, many of whom do not fit the stereotypical profile of people we'd expect to have a bad outcome with COVID. They are young. They are fit. They are high school sports stars, adults in their prime with no previous health problems or preexisting conditions, professional athletes, special operations military personnel, and doctors themselves. They cannot make sense of their body's rollercoaster reaction to COVID. Although women seem to be more at risk for long-haul COVID, we cannot dismiss the outliers to that pattern who are part of this conversation and whose experience will add to our knowledge and library of COVID medicine.

My advice to anyone suffering from long-haul COVID is to find one of these post-COVID clinics near you that bring together specialists across the board — pulmonary, cardiology, and neurology. Make it a "family affair" in medicine and at home. This takes a multidisciplinary group approach to cover the panoply of syndromes. Survivor Corps (SurvivorCorps.com) is a great gateway for resources. It is worth noting that many long-haulers have found relief through vaccination, which is great news and a clue to what is causing the symptoms to persist in the first place. For everyone else, it also provides another reason to get vaccinated and stay on top of possible booster shots in the future.

Speaking of booster shots, if needed, I won't hesitate to get one to keep my COVID immunity up to speed with the globe-trotting variants. COVID will continue to chase us, but we can chase life with science on our side.

CHAPTER 9
F: FIGHT FOR THE FUTURE OF US

YOUR HEALTH DEPENDS ON EVERYONE ELSE'S AROUND THE WORLD

Over the past twenty years, I have covered nearly every outbreak, epidemic, and pandemic in the world. When SARS erupted in 2003, I was in Iraq embedded with the US Marine medical unit known as the Devil Docs. Even during a war, the story of what was happening in China at that time broke through and frightened people. Sitting outside our tents with gunfire in the distance, I remember the Marines asking me how concerned they should be about the virus. As you know by now, SARS ended up being relatively rare, with fewer than ten thousand cases diagnosed in the entire world. Many may forget, however, that the case fatality rate was about 10 percent, which means for every 100 people who contracted the virus, 10 died from the resulting disease (the case fatality rate is the number of confirmed deaths divided by the number of confirmed cases). It is hard to conceive what impact COVID-19 would've had if it was similarly deadly.*

Two years after the SARS outbreak, I was in Thailand, Laos, and Indonesia covering H5N1, the avian flu. Details were sparse when we arrived during the 2005 holidays and stayed over the new year into 2006. There were just a few dozen cases, but the fatality rate was already well above 40 percent and would continue to climb. Back then, a frequent guest during my live reporting was Dr. Anthony Fauci. "This is the one

* COVID's case fatality rate is constantly changing and differs throughout the world, depending on public health measures and how the virus is behaving in a community. Clearly, we've learned that case fatality rates rise for older individuals and those with preexisting conditions. Interestingly, COVID became the third-leading cause of death for individuals forty years old and over in 2020, with an overall annual mortality rate of 325 deaths per 100,000 individuals, behind only cancer and heart disease. In addition, for individuals forty years old and over, the case fatality rate for COVID was greater than the case fatality rate for motor vehicle accidents.

that keeps me up at night," he had told me back then. A highly deadly flu that was also very contagious. Fortuitously, neither SARS nor H5N1 spread easily around the world.

Three years after that, in 2009, another flu virus started to spread from a small region of central Mexico. It was called H1N1 or swine flu. (The term *swine flu* is a misnomer; this strain is made up of several different components, including swine but also avian parts.) Five-year-old Edgar Hernandez was believed to be patient zero, first identified in a story I did for CNN as we traveled through Mexico with a group of disease detectives. Unlike SARS and H5N1, the swine flu was very contagious, and 60 million people in the United States were believed to have been infected between April 2009 and April 2010. The case fatality rate, though, was much lower: 0.02 percent. There were more than 270,000 hospitalizations and around 12,000 people died of that flu. Although the disease wasn't that deadly, I can tell you from personal experience, it was awful.

Throughout all of my coverage and travels to hot zones, I stayed disease free until September 2009. I was once again in the Middle East, this time covering the conflict in Afghanistan. It started as a cough for me.

That wasn't unusual: We were in the desert, and dust was constantly being kicked up into the air. But my cough was different. It hurt — a stinging pain that made me wince and immediately hope that I didn't have to cough again anytime soon. I thought I might have a fever, but of course, I was in the middle of covering a war in Afghanistan, and the conditions were, well, hot. So maybe it was that. Problem was, the next day I was feeling worse. I woke up in my dusty desert tent and tried to step out of my sleeping bag. Two steps later, I hit the deck. My body simply could not hold me up. I was light-headed and freezing cold, even though it was already over 100 degrees outside at that early hour of the morning.

I was nauseated, and my entire body ached. I tried to explain away my symptoms with lots of different excuses. You don't sleep much while covering a war. My bulletproof jacket didn't fit perfectly and was very heavy. Maybe I had what the Marines referred to as the Kandahar Krud. It turned out to be none of those things. I remember looking over at my cameraman, Scottie McWhinnie. He looked absolutely awful too. He was wearing a scarf on his head and it was drenched in sweat. He was coughing so loudly and frequently that I was starting to worry about him — and about myself. We each had it, whatever "it" was. I made a command decision: As a physician reporter in a war zone, I was going to get us medical care.[1] That prompted a visit to a battlefield hospital, not as reporters this time but as patients. There wasn't much they could do for us, except confirm that it was in fact H1N1 and pump us full of IV fluids.

This was the sickest I have ever been and, in the days it took me to recover, I lost fourteen pounds. My wife looked at me horrified when I finally arrived home. It took a lot of convincing a few years later when I told her I was thinking about flying to another hot zone — this time to cover the hemorrhagic fever Ebola, which ended up being one of the most profound experiences of all.

Spring 2014
It took only moments to feel the impact of what was happening. My crew and I had just landed in Conakry, the capital of Guinea in West Africa. In the fields right outside the airport, a young woman was in tears. She started to wail and shout in Susu, one of the forty languages spoken in this tiny country of 12 million people that is also one of the poorest places in the world. The

gathered crowd became silent and listened intently. The young man sitting next to me quietly translated, although I already had my suspicions. He told me the woman's husband had died of Ebola, and then he quickly ushered us away.

Ebola rarely made it out of the remote forested areas of Africa, but there was growing concern about it reaching populous areas, including where I'd just touched down, an international airport. Guinea's foreign minister initially said that the West African country had brought the spread of the deadly Ebola virus under control after more than a hundred people had died. When I asked doctors on the ground about the risk of Ebola breaching the gates of the country and making a global escape, however, they had split opinions. Several told me the concern was real but unlikely. Most patients with Ebola came from small villages in the forest and were unlikely to fly on international trips, they told me. Furthermore, they didn't think Ebola would spread widely in a Western country like the United States; our medical expertise and our culture — not touching the dead — would prevent it. Others weren't so sure, and no one wanted to test that theory.

With Ebola, there is an incubation period

of two to twenty-one days, the range of time it takes to develop symptoms after someone has been exposed. With an international airport close by, that means you could be on the other side of the world before you develop the headache, fever, fatigue, and joint pain that make up the early symptoms of an Ebola infection. The diarrhea, rash, and bleeding come later. Hiccups are a particularly grave sign with Ebola. It means your diaphragm, which allows you to breathe, is starting to get irritated.

Like COVID, there is a lot we have learned about Ebola, and it scares us almost as much as what we don't know. We do know that Ebola, a simple virus with a small genome, is a swift, effective, and bloody killer — the contagion of horror movies.[2] The mortality rate is higher than 50 percent, and in some outbreaks, it reaches 90 percent. Ebola appears to kill in a clever way. Early on, it strategically disarms your immune system, allowing the virus to replicate unchecked until it invades organs throughout your body. It convinces your blood to clot in overdrive, but only inside your blood vessels. While those blood vessels choke up, the rest of your body starts to ooze because the clotting mechanisms are all busy. You start to hemorrhage on the outside of your body. Your nose and eyes bleed; you start to bruise, and there is no clotting when you puncture your skin. But it is the bleeding you don't see, the bleeding on the inside, that causes even more catastrophic problems. Many patients die of shock within an average of ten days.

Yet despite the real danger, Ebola is not easy to "catch." To become infected, you generally need to spend extended time with someone who is gravely ill and come into contact with his or her infected body fluids. That's why family members and health care workers are the most likely to get sick. With some infections, including COVID, you can shed and spread the virus long before you get ill. That's not the case with Ebola. Only after you are sick and feverish do you become contagious. However, it only takes a minuscule amount to infect and kill. A microscopic droplet of blood or saliva on your bare hand could enter through a break in your skin. And whether you realize it or not, we all have breaks in our skin. After being on the ground for a few days, I realized it was only a matter of time before Ebola would breach the gates of Africa.

A few months later, as the outbreaks continued to rage in West Africa, Ebola landed in the United States. The virus first arrived via US missionaries flown here for treatment over the summer. It was also unwittingly imported by a forty-two-year-old Liberian tourist named Thomas Eric Duncan, who flew from Liberia to Texas with the virus and later died in Dallas. Two nurses who treated Duncan contracted Ebola on American soil, and both recovered. We all heard about these cases in the media, and rallied for the infected. Overall, eleven people were successfully treated for Ebola in the United States during the 2014 epidemic that originated in West Africa.

This is a crucial point, and brings us to our last lesson. None of the patients who contracted the virus in America died, and yet more than one in two perished in Africa. Although the virus doesn't discriminate, your survival depends not only on the country but also the zip code of where you were infected. All of the survivors in the United States had one thing in common: They were rushed to two of the country's four hospitals, including my own at Emory University, that had been preparing for years to treat a highly infectious disease such as Ebola.

That wasn't an option during the COVID pandemic and as a result we witnessed awful discrepancies in outcomes across the country. Ebola is probably never going to spread in the United States as it can elsewhere because it's just not the kind of virus that can gain the upper hand in our system. But a germ like COVID? It demonstrated how quickly it could move, and how badly prepared we were to manage the damage equitably, both at home and as citizens of the world. COVID also showed how little we understand the public health adage I first heard in Africa: An outbreak anywhere in the world is an outbreak everywhere in the world. Remote corners of the world may as well be in our backyards. Until we fill the gaps and close the divides globally and nationally, a pathogen like COVID could be as horrific and devastating a menace as Ebola.

This is why we each have an obligation to make sure we help prevent outbreaks in distant lands. In an ideal scenario, the most vulnerable to a disease would be vaccinated first, no matter where they live. Instead we find ourselves vaccinating a person every second in wealthy countries while some countries haven't received any vaccines at all. As of spring 2021, the vast majority of all vaccines have gone to high-income countries (reflecting 16 percent of the world's population) while less than 1 percent have gone to the low-income tier.[3]

INDIA'S SECOND DEADLY SURGE IS A CAUTIONARY TALE

On April 23, 2021, I was feeling more optimistic than I had in a long time. My wife and I even went out to dinner with a couple of friends at a local restaurant, dining outside. Admittedly, it was a bit socially awkward, given it was the first time we had done this in more than a year. But as we lowered our masks and saw smiling faces, it felt really good, almost normal. We gossiped about what was happening in the neighborhood, swapped some good quarantine stories, and even made plans to do it again soon. For the first time, the future didn't feel blank to me, as it had for so long, stuck in my sensory-deprived basement.

I woke up the next morning to shattering news: A beloved uncle had suddenly and very unexpectedly died of COVID in New Delhi, India. He had become ill the previous Monday, was hospitalized on Tuesday, and died Thursday. The cremation was scheduled the next day. It was so swift that it felt like a death from a traumatic accident as opposed to from an infectious disease. This particular uncle was a favorite among the dozens of our Gupta cousins. He was the natural storyteller, always wore a smile, and was also the most permissive of all the elders — sneaking us drinks at family weddings. He was a perfectly healthy man in his early seventies until COVID claimed him.

It was also particularly shocking because after riding a long but mostly contained wave of COVID in 2020, India looked to be in great shape in early 2021. The second most populous country after China, India is home to one out of every six human beings on the planet. In the first week of March, its health minister declared that it was in the "endgame." But by mid-March a devastating second surge took the country by surprise, and cases climbed sharply until they hit the world's highest single-day count since the pandemic began — more than 400,000 new infections, beating a previous record set by the United States with 300,310 new cases on January 2. The case counts and deaths were likely massively underreported.

Hospitals ran out of space, oxygen and antivirals disappeared, and the descent into crisis led to massive cremation sites being created out of parking lots. Reasons for the surge included a vacuum of leadership in the central government and an exhausted public eager to let its guard down after an

Daily New Confirmed COVID-19 Cases per Million People Shown is the rolling seven-day average. The number of confirmed cases is lower than the number of actual cases; the main reason for that is limited testing.

Source: Johns Hopkins University CSSE COVID-19 Data[4]

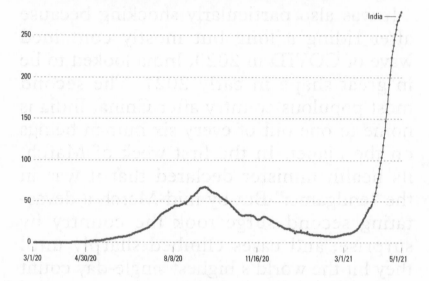

intense lockdown in the first wave that crushed their economy. Leaders did little to discourage public gatherings, allowing a massive weeks-long Hindu pilgrimage to proceed with millions of attendees traveling across numerous states. At the same time, political rallies attracted large unmasked crowds and became superspreader events. New, stickier, and more contagious variants were born that were more lethal, deepening the death toll. Experts' warnings about a potential second wave had gone unheeded. The country, once a model for its pandemic response, suddenly found itself at the forefront of the news. People around the world watched, wondering what it all meant for them. There was some good news: The existing vaccines were still protective against the emerging variants in India, but only if you were lucky enough to get one.

India happens to be one of the largest producers of vaccines in the world, but it exported much of its supply before inoculating its own people. By the time the second surge took off and people needed medical help, it was too late to mitigate and contain the virus. Barely 3 percent of India's population had been fully vaccinated, and only 9.2 percent of people had received at least one dose when the second wave hit.[6] My uncle, who would have been in the first group of eligible people in the United States, had not yet had access to the vaccine.

My parents, raised in India, were particularly disturbed by this. They had received the first shot of their vaccine at the end of December 2020. My mom, one of the most determined people I know, had found that her local county library had three hundred doses of the COVID vaccine available and would start immunizing at 9:00 a.m. on December 29. She grabbed my dad and camped out in front of the library starting at 1:30 a.m. It was as if she were waiting for tickets to a Grateful Dead concert! They were eventually given numbers 288 and 289 and happily sent me pictures of their vaccine cards later that morning. By May 10, my three girls had the vaccine authorized for them and were among the first very enthusiastic customers in their age group. We couldn't help but wonder: If my uncle had been a resident in the United States, would he still be living today? And my dad wondered aloud what would have happened to him if he had never left India.

HOPE IN A HURRY

Pandemics unmask who we really are — our morals, our values, our ethics, our humanity. They test us in ways that nothing else can. But despite the losses and hardships we've all endured over the pandemic so far, there have been moments when the best of our humanity has come through. People I've talked to have shared beautiful stories of rekindling old friendships, connecting better with loved ones during lockdown, spending more time in the kitchen and garden, learning new skills and finding fresh hobbies, reaffirming their sense of purpose in work or perhaps seeking new purpose in a different job, feeling a greater awareness of culture and community, and overall being more conscious of the fragility of life. I encourage all of you to try to take this opportunity to reflect about what changes from the pandemic you might want to make permanent and which habits you are most eager to abandon.

I am an eternal optimist and trust we will continue to rise to whatever occasions await us in the future. More than one hundred years ago, the pandemic of 1918 killed nearly 200,000 Americans in October alone.[7] The antimasking campaigns were relentless. The volume of people arrested for refusing to wear masks so overburdened the court system that public health authorities stopped making arrests. The case numbers started to climb again after Thanksgiving, partially blamed on Armistice Day celebrations for the end of World War I and relaxed restrictions over the holidays as people grew tired of pandemic life. But we all know that viruses don't take a vacation. In December, news headlines said Santa Claus was "Down with the Flu" as schools closed and health officials ordered department stores to dispense with "Santa Claus programs."[8] By January, the country was fully engulfed in the pandemic's third wave, and it would not subside until the summer of 1919.

A lot has happened in the past century. Since the Great Influenza, we've gained the Internet and smartphones, extraordinary medical technology, and a greater understanding about diseases and ways to treat them. The COVID crisis finally propelled mRNA vaccines across the finish line, which will prove to be a powerful tool throughout many fields of medicine. But the pandemic also took us down to the studs of what life is about. As my wife tells me, "It'll be a bad scar that still aches sometimes because we'll always still feel bad about all the lives lost to this pandemic, but we'll learn and move forward and still grow and develop in a way that helps us in the future."

I know I have.

ACKNOWLEDGMENTS

We have always shared our beautiful Goldilocks planet with creatures big and small, and yet we are still learning to dance with them. Our moves are sometimes clumsy, and we too often step on our partners' toes. We infringe on their space, strip away their habitat, and needlessly take their lives. There is a best way to live, where we give as much as we take, protect our precious resources, and respect our Earthmates. It is possible to live well and do the perfect tango at the same time.

Since the beginning of 2020, I have spent countless hours with the elite of public health, policy, and prediction. They live audacious lives, believing we can become pandemic proof, and rid ourselves of the existential threat pathogens pose to mankind. They are the dance instructors we all need, and they inspired me to write this book. The medical team at CNN are truly the best on the planet, and helped guide my thinking on this book. Ben Tinker, Amanda Sealy, Nadia Kounang, Michael Nedelman, Tia Miller, and Jessica Small have all been completely immersed in telling the story of COVID accurately and fairly.

Priscilla Painton is blessed with many talents, but it is her gift of clarity that is a blessing to her writers. Having had an extraordinary experience working on *Keep Sharp* with Priscilla, I wondered if it was a fluke. Now with two data points, it is looking like a trend. I am looking forward to collecting more evidence.

A book like this is only possible because of the team of dreamers who make the pages come to life and then tell the world about it. Yvette Grant, Megan Hogan, and Hana Park, thank you for your editorial guidance. Julia Prosser, Stephen Bedford, Elizabeth Gay Herman, and Elise Ringo, thank you for finding the best ways to connect *WWC* to the audience. Jackie Seow and Paul Dippolito, the book is a work of art because of you. While I will never get used to having my picture on the cover of a book, I am grateful for your diligence and brilliance. A book about a pandemic should be available all over the world, and because of the hard work of Marie Florio, it will be.

Great teams start with great leaders. Dana Canedy, I am appreciative of all your support. Jonathan Karp, our conversations remain some of my favorite of all. I remain mesmerized by your ability to toggle so effortlessly between pandemics and politics, sports, and Springsteen. Tremendously grateful for your warmth and willingness to welcome me to the family.

Every time I am lucky enough to spend some time talking to the world's greatest lawyer, Bob Barnett, I walk away more informed and more inspired. I am still not certain why he included me on his list of clients, ranging from presidents to the pope, but being a friend of Bob is one of my life's greatest honors.

And Kristin Loberg. An acknowledgment seems hardly enough to best describe our wonderful burgeoning partnership, facilitated by the indefatigable and supportive Bonnie Solow. For the past year, we rode side by side in a speeding car, burning rubber, and even accelerating through the turns. We did it because we knew it was important. When my gas tank started to run low, you were there cheering me on, keeping me awake, and reminding me of the mission. Your light burns bright, Kristin, and I get to be one of the lucky ones, basking in the glow. I will forever be indebted to you, my dear friend.

NOTES

Author's Note

The selected list of notes to accompany statements made in the book became a tome in itself due to the volume of sources and scientific literature I could have cited. Below is a snapshot of resources that will at least help lead you to more sources and provide a launchpad for further inquiry. Some of the stories in the book were reported on widely by the media, and when it came to the details of COVID victims, either names and identifying materials were changed or their stories had already been made public. I trust you can find a wellspring of references and evidence yourself online with just a few taps of the keyboard, assuming you visit reputable sites that post fact-checked, credible information that's been vetted by experts. This is especially important when it comes to matters of health and medicine.

As we all know, the COVID-19 pandemic

remains a dynamic event with its growing body of knowledge evolving daily. Unintended omissions in the book are indeed possible as a result, but I've done my very best to present the most credible, science-backed information with clarity, transparency, and endless fact-checking. Some of my content is based on my own interactions both in my professional work as a journalist and in personal conversations with colleagues and people who were familiar with the matters and openly shared their insights.

Introduction: A "Pneumonia of Unknown Origin"

1 See "China Investigates Respiratory Illness Outbreak Sickening 27," AP News, December 31, 2019, https://apnews.com/article/wuhan-health-international-news-china-severe-acute-respiratory-syndrome-00c78d1974410d96fe031f67edbd86ec. Several timelines of the pandemic's development have been published online. You can access these just by searching for "COVID timeline."

2 See Michael C. Bender and Rebecca Ballhaus, "A Landmark White House Move Left States to Secure Medical Equipment Themselves, Causing Problems that Still

432

Haven't Abated," *Wall Street Journal,* August 31, 2020, https://www.wsj.com/articles/how-trump-sowed-covid-supply-chaos-try-getting-it-yourselves-1159889 3051.

3 See Elizabeth Arias, Betzaida Tejada-Vera, and Farida Ahmad, "Provisional Life Expectancy Estimates for January through June, 2020," *Vital Statistics Rapid Release,* Report no. 10, February 2021, https://www.cdc.gov/nchs/data/vsrr/VSRR10-508.pdf.

4 See Xixing Li, Weina Cui, and Fuzhen Zhang, "Who Was the First Doctor to Report the COVID-19 Outbreak in Wuhan, China?" *Journal of Nuclear Medicine* 61, no. 6 (June 2020): 782–783, doi: 10.2967/jnumed.120.247262. Epub 2020 Apr 17.

5 See "Novel Coronavirus — Thailand (ex-China)," Disease Outbreak News, January 14, 2020, World Health Organization, https://www.who.int/csr/don/14-january-2020-novel-coronavirus-thailand-ex-china/en/.

6 See Keri N. Althoff et al., "Antibodies to SARS-CoV-2 in All of Us Research Program Participants, January 2–March 18, 2020," *Clinical Infectious Diseases* (June 2021): ciab519, doi: 10.1093/cid/ciab519.

7 See Jamie Gangel, Jeremy Herb, and Elizabeth Stuart, " 'Play It Down': Trump Admits to Concealing the True Threat of Coronavirus in New Woodward Book," CNN, September 9, 2020, https://www.cnn.com/2020/09/09/politics/bob-woodward-rage-book-trump-coronavirus/index.html. Also see Bob Woodward, *Rage* (New York: Simon & Schuster, 2020).

8 See "Secretary Azar Declares Public Health Emergency for United States for 2019 Novel Coronavirus," HHS Press Office, January 31, 2020, https://www.hhs.gov/about/news/2020/01/31/secretary-azar-declares-public-health-emergency-us-2019-novel-coronavirus.html.

9 See Jane C. Hu, "Covid's Cassandra: The Swift, Complicated Rise of Eric Feigl-Ding," *Undark,* November 25, 2020, https://undark.org/2020/11/25/complicated-rise-of-eric-feigl-ding/.

10 See Maxime Taquet et al., "6-month Neurological and Psychiatric Outcomes in 236, 379 Survivors of COVID-19: A Retrospective Cohort Study Using Electronic Health Records," *Lancet Psychiatry* 8, no. 5 (May 2021): 416–427, doi: 10.1016/S2215-0366(21)00084-5. Epub 2021 Apr 6.

11 Maya Angelou was linked to this saying in 2003, but reports have since emerged to show that the line could have originated from a 1971 collection called *Richard Evans' Quote Book* and been ascribed to Carl W. Buehner, a high-level official in the Mormon church who said, "They may forget what you said — but they will never forget how you made them feel."

12 See Sanjay Gupta, "The Big One Is Coming, and It's Going to Be a Flu Pandemic," CNN, November 7, 2018, https://www.cnn.com/2017/04/07/health/flu-pandemic-sanjay-gupta/index.html.

13 See Johns Hopkins University Bloomberg School of Public Health, "Global Health Security Index Finds Gaps in Preparedness for Epidemics and Pandemics: Even High-income Countries Are Found Lacking and Score Only in the Average Range of Preparedness," *Science-Daily,* http://www.sciencedaily.com/releases/2019/10/191024115022.htm (accessed June 2, 2021).

14 See Steven H. Woolf, Derek A. Chapman, and Jong Hyung Lee, "COVID-19 as the Leading Cause of Death in the United States," *JAMA* 325, no. 2 (December 2020): 123–124, doi: 10.1001/jama.2020.24865.

15 See "Bird Flu: Russia Detects First Case of H5N8 Bird Flu in Humans," BBC News, February 20, 2021, https://www.bbc.com/news/world-europe-56140270.

16 See Vivian Wang, "A Man in China Is Found to Have H10N3 Bird Flu, a Reminder of a Continued 'Concern for Pandemic Flu'," *New York Times,* June 2, 2021, https://www.nytimes.com/2021/06/02/world/asia/h10n3-bird-flu.html.

17 See Peter M. Sandman, "A Severe Pandemic Is Not Overdue — It's Not When But If," Center for Infectious Disease Research and Policy, News & Perspective, February 22, 2007, https://www.cidrap.umn.edu/news-perspective/2007/02/severe-pandemic-not-overdue-its-not-when-if.

Chapter 1: Postmortem

1 See "What It's Like to Lose Someone to Covid-19," *New York Times,* March 5, 2021, https://www.nytimes.com/interactive/2021/03/05/us/covid-deaths.html.

2 See Dr. Sanjay Gupta, "The Pandemic Has Become a Humanitarian Disaster in the United States," CNN, November 13, 2020, https://www.cnn.com/2020/11/13/health/coronavirus-humanitarian-disaster-

gupta/index.html.

3 See Olga Khazan, "A Failure of Empathy Led to 200,000 Deaths. It Has Deep Roots," *Atlantic,* September 22, 2020, https://www.theatlantic.com/politics/archive/2020/09/covid-death-toll-us-empathy-elderly/616379/.

4 See "DHS Issues Supplemental Instructions for Inbound Flights with Individuals Who Have Been In China," News Archive from the Department of Homeland Security, February 2, 2020, https://www.dhs.gov/news/2020/02/02/dhs-issues-supplemental-instructions-inbound-flights-individuals-who-have-been-china.

5 See Patricia Mazzei, "A Family's Search for Answers: Did Their Brother Die of Covid?" *New York Times,* March 7, 2021, https://www.nytimes.com/2021/03/07/us/florida-family-coronavirus-death.html.

6 See Charles A. Downs et al., "COVID Symptoms, Symptom Clusters, and Predictors for Becoming a Long-Hauler: Looking for Clarity in the Haze of the Pandemic," preprint, *medRxiv,* posted March 5, 2021, doi: 10.1101/2021.03.03.21252086.

7 See Mark Honigsbaum and Lakshmi Krishnan, "Taking Pandemic Sequelae

Seriously: From the Russian Influenza to COVID-19 Long-haulers," *Lancet* 396, no. 10260 (October 2020): 1389–1391, doi: 10.1016/S0140-6736(20)32134-6. Epub 2020 Oct 12.

8 Ibid.

9 My one-on-one interviews with six of the members of Trump's coronavirus task force were done in the development of a special report for CNN called "COVID WAR — The Pandemic Doctors Speak Out" that aired on March 28, 2021. The recorded conversations amounted to hours of tape. Many of the quotes and paraphrased material in this book came from those interactions. See Dr. Sanjay Gupta, "Autopsy of a Pandemic: 6 Doctors at the Center of the US Covid-19 Response," CNN, March 26, 2021, https://www.cnn.com/2021/03/26/health/covid-war-doctors-sanjay-gupta/index.html.

10 See Fernanda Santos, "Life, Death, and Grief in Los Angeles," *New York Times Magazine,* March 2, 2021, https://www.nytimes.com/interactive/2021/03/02/magazine/covid-la-county-hospitals-black-latino-residents.html.

11 Ibid.

12 To view cases and deaths from COVID worldwide by country as the numbers

changed throughout the pandemic, use the interactive dashboard provided by the Center for Systems Science and Engineering (CSSE) at Johns Hopkins University at https://github.com/CSSEGISandData/COVID-19. Also see E. Dong, H. Du, and L. Gardner, "An Interactive Web-based Dashboard to Track COVID-19 in Real Time," *Lancet Infectious Diseases* 20, no. 5 (2020): 533–534, doi: 10.1016/S1473-3099(20)30120-1.

13 See Matthew Mosk, "George W. Bush in 2005: 'If We Wait for a Pandemic to Appear, It Will Be Too Late to Prepare'," ABC News, April 5, 2020, https://abcnews.go.com/Politics/george-bush-2005-wait-pandemic-late-prepare/story?id=699790 13. Also see John M. Barry, *The Great Influenza* (New York: Viking Penguin, 2004).

14 Ibid. According to the media's reports, Tom Bossert used the word *obsessed* to describe Bush's response. Bossert had worked in the Bush White House and went on to serve as a homeland security adviser in the Trump administration.

15 Ibid.

16 See "Crimson Contagion 2019 Functional Exercise Key Findings," US Department of Health and Human Services, Of-

fice of the Assistant Secretary for Preparedness and Response (October 2019), https://int.nyt.com/data/document helper/6824-2019-10-key-findings-and-after/05bd797500ea55be0724/optimized/full.pdf. Also see David E. Sanger, Eric Lipton, Eileen Sullivan, and Michael Crowley, "Before Virus Outbreak, a Cascade of Warnings Went Unheeded," *New York Times,* March 19, 2020, https://www.nytimes.com/2020/03/19/us/politics/trump-coronavirus-outbreak.html.

17 See Susan Davis, Claudia Grisales, and Kelsey Snell, "Senate Passes $2 Trillion Coronavirus Relief Package," NPR, March 25, 2020, https://www.npr.org/2020/03/25/818881845/senate-reaches-historic-deal-on-2t-coronavirus-economic-rescue-package.

18 See Maggie Haberman, "Trump Admits Downplaying the Virus Knowing It Was 'Deadly Stuff,' " *New York Times,* September 9, 2020, https://www.nytimes.com/2020/09/09/us/politics/woodward-trump-bookvirus.html.

19 The reality distortion field was often used to describe how Steve Jobs would influence his employees at Apple. According to Walter Isaacson's chronicle of the Apple icon in his biography (*Steve Jobs:*

440

The Exclusive Biography), Jobs had learned about the reality distortion field — a term used to describe how someone can influence people and convince them of almost anything with a mix of characteristics including charm, bravado, hyperbole, and of course persistence.

20 Several reprints of Defoe's *Journal of the Plague Year* are available online for free or purchase. Here's one place to read it: https://www.gutenberg.org/files/376/376-h/376-h.htm.

21 See E. Dong, H. Du, and L. Gardner, "An Interactive Web-based Dashboard to Track COVID-19 in Real Time," *Lancet Infectious Diseases* 20 no. 5 (2020): 533–534. doi: 10.1016/S1473-3099(20)30120-1. Also see the interactive dashboard provided by the Center for Systems Science and Engineering (CSSE) at Johns Hopkins University at https://github.com/CSSEGISandData/COVID-19.

22 Ibid.

23 See Azeem Majeed et al., "Can the UK Emulate the South Korean Approach to Covid-19?" *BMJ* 369 (May 2020): m2084, doi: 10.1136/bmj.m2084. Also see Daejoong Lee, Kyungmoo Heo, and Yongseok Seo, "COVID-19 in South Korea: Lessons for Developing Countries," *World Develop-*

ment 135 (November 2020): 105057, doi: 10.1016/j.worlddev.2020.105057. Epub 2020 Jun 28.

24 See the Centers for Disease Control and Prevention's data and statistics on obesity at https://www.cdc.gov/obesity/data/adult.html.

25 See Alireza Bolourian and Zahra Mojtahedi, "COVID-19 and Flu Pandemics Follow a Pattern: A Possible Cross-immunity in the Pandemic Origin and Graver Disease in Farther Regions," *Archives of Medical Research* 52, no. 2 (February 2021): 240–241, doi: 10.1016/j.arcmed.2020.10.012. Epub 2020 Oct 17.

26 Jose Mateus et al., "Selective and Cross-reactive SARS-CoV-2 T Cell Epitopes in Unexposed Humans," *Science* 370, no. 6512 (October 2020): 89–94, doi: 10.1126/science.abd3871. Epub 2020 Aug 4.

27 See Dr. Sanjay Gupta, "The United States' One-year Coronavirus Checkup," CNN, January 21, 2021, http://lite.cnn.com/en/article/h_0e1a2ddf94eeb132a 5b deecdda84a602.

28 See Sen Pei, Sasikiran Kandula, and Jeffrey Shaman, "Differential Effects of Intervention Timing on COVID-19 Spread in the United States," *Science Ad-*

vances 6, no. 49 (December 2020): eabd6370, https://advances.sciencemag .org/content/6/49/eabd6370.

29 In addition to sharing these insights with me personally in a formal interview, Dr. Birx also made these statements on *Face the Nation* with Margaret Brennan on February 24, 2021. The transcript is available here: https://www.cbsnews.com/news/ transcript-deborah-birx-on-face-the-nation-january-24-2021/.

30 Several media outlets called February 2020 "The Lost Month": See Marshall Cohen, Tara Subramaniam, and Christopher Hickey, "The Lost Month," CNN, April 18, 2020, https://www.cnn.com/ interactive/2020/04/politics/trump-covid-response-annotation/.

31 The National Commission on Terrorist Attacks Upon the United States (also known as the 9-11 Commission) report is available online at https://9-11commission .gov/report/.

32 See Gupta, "The United States' One-year Coronavirus Checkup."

33 See Sanjay Gupta, "Why CNN Is Calling the Novel Coronavirus Outbreak a Pandemic," CNN, March 9, 2020, https:// www.cnn.com/2020/03/09/health/corona virus-pandemic-gupta/index.html.

34 See the CDC's resource page on pandemics at https://www.cdc.gov/flu/pandemic-resources/index.htm.

35 See the transcript of Dr. Messonnier's briefing at https://www.cdc.gov/media/releases/2020/t0225-cdc-telebriefing-covid-19.html.

36 Ibid.

37 See Pam Belluck and Noah Weiland, "C.D.C. Officials Warn of Coronavirus Outbreaks in the U.S.," *New York Times,* February 25, 2020, https://www.nytimes.com/2020/02/25/health/coronavirus-us.html.

38 See Gupta, "Why CNN Is Calling the Novel Coronavirus Outbreak a Pandemic."

Chapter 2: Multisystem Organ Failure

1 See the *New York Times*'s reports on the Red Dawn emails at www.nytimes.com. Also see Eric Lipton, "The 'Red Dawn' Emails: 8 Key Exchanges on the Faltering Response to the Coronavirus," *New York Times,* April 11, 2020, https://www.nytimes.com/2020/04/11/us/politics/coronavirus-red-dawn-emails-trump.html. Some of the emails were also reported by Kaiser Health News at https://khn.org/news/red-

dawn-breaking-bad-officials-warned-about-safety-gear-shortfall-early-on-emails-show/.

2 See Bob Woodward, *Rage* (New York: Simon & Schuster, 2020).

3 See Matthew Pottinger's full interview on *Face the Nation* with Margaret Brenner on February 21, 2021, at https://www.cbs news.com/news/transcript-matt-potting er-on-face-the-nation-february-21-2021/.

4 The exact words used by George Gao could not be confirmed. This statement captures Bob Redfield's best recollection of the conversation when I interviewed him in February 2021.

5 See Michael R. Gordon, Warren P. Strobel, and Drew Hinshaw, "Intelligence on Sick Staff at Wuhan Lab Fuels Debate on Covid-19 Origin," *Wall Street Journal*, May 23, 2021, https://www.wsj.com/articles/intelligence-on-sick-staff-at-wuhan-lab-fuels-debate-on-covid-19-origin-11621796228.

6 Ibid. Also see Jeremy Page, Drew Hinshaw, and Betsy McKay, "In Hunt for Covid-19 Origin, Patient Zero Points to Second Wuhan Market," *Wall Street Journal*, February 26, 2021, https://www.wsj.com/articles/n-hunt-for-covid-19-origin-patient-zero-points-to-second-wuhan-

market-11614335404?mod=article_in line.

7 See the Red Dawn emails, notably the one from James A. Lawler on January 28, 2020, at https://www.nytimes.com/2020/04/11/us/politics/coronavirus-red-dawn-emails-trump.html.

8 Takuya Yamagishi et al., "Descriptive Study of COVID-19 Outbreak among Passengers and Crew on *Diamond Princess* Cruise Ship, Yokohama Port, Japan, 20 January to 9 February 2020," *Euro-surveillance* 25, no. 23 (June 2020): 2000272, doi: 10.2807/1560-7917.ES .2020.25.23.2000272.

9 See the CDC's media statement, "Cruise Ship No Sail Order Extended through September 2020," on July 16, 2020, at https://www.cdc.gov/media/releases/2020/s0716-cruise-ship-no-sail-order.html.

10 See John S. Brownstein et al., "Analysis of Hospital Traffic and Search Engine Data in Wuhan China Indicates Early Disease Activity in the Fall of 2019," (2020). The file can be downloaded at http://nrs.harvard.edu/urn-3:HUL.InstRe pos:42669767.

11 For a summary of the main beats to these exchanges from my series of interviews that aired on CNN on March 28,

2021 ("COVID WAR — The Pandemic Doctors Speak Out"), see Sheryl Gay Stolberg, "Covid-19: Birx Lashes Trump's Pandemic Response and Says Deaths Could Have Been 'Decreased Substantially,' " *New York Times,* April 30, 2021, https://www.nytimes.com/live/2021/03/28/world/covid-vaccine-coronavirus-cases. See Dr. Sanjay Gupta, "Autopsy of a Pandemic: 6 Doctors at the Center of the US Covid-19 Response," CNN, March 26, 2021, https://www.cnn.com/2021/03/26/health/covid-war-doctors-sanjay-gupta/index.html. Also see https://edition.cnn.com/health/live-news/covid-pandemic-doctors-cnn-special/index.html.

12 See Erin Banco and Asawin Suebsaeng, "Team Trump Pushes CDC to Revise Down Its COVID Death Counts," *Daily Beast,* May 13, 2020, https://www.thedailybeast.com/team-trump-pushes-cdc-to-dial-down-covid-death-counts?ref=home.

13 To see examples of these headlines, see "Fact Check: 94% of Individuals with Additional Causes of Death Still Had COVID-19," by Reuters Staff on September 3, 2020, https://www.reuters.com/article/uk-factcheck-94-percent-covid-among-caus/fact-check-94-of-individuals-

with-additional-causes-of-death-still-had-covid-19-idUSKBN25U2IO.

14 See Steven H. Woolf et al., "Excess Deaths From COVID-19 and Other Causes in the US, March 1, 2020, to January 2, 2021," *JAMA* 325, no. 17 (April 2021): 1786–1789, doi: 10.1001/jama .2021.5199.

Chapter 3: Snakes

1 See Sanjay Gupta, "Dr. Sanjay Gupta Remembers 'Giant' of Neurosurgery Who Separated Conjoined Twins," CNN, March 31, 2020, https://www.cnn.com/2020/03/31/health/neurosurgeon-goodrich-tribute-conjoined-twins/index.html.

2 See Mallory Simon and Melissa Dunst Lipman, "Charlotte Figi, the Girl Who Inspired a CBD Movement, Has Died at Age 13," CNN, April 9, 2020, https://www.cnn.com/2020/04/08/health/charlotte-figi-cbd-marijuana-dies/index.html.

3 Plenty of online destinations can provide you with a basic course on viruses, from where they come from and their history to their biology, how they behave and act differently. I recommend checking out papers published by the National Center for

Biotechnology Information, which is part of the United States National Library of Medicine, a branch of the National Institutes of Health (https://www.ncbi.nlm.nih.gov/). Sal Khan maintains a terrific set of videos you can also watch as part of his Khan Academy (https://www.khanacademy.org/).

4 See Ann C. Gregory et al., "Marine DNA Viral Macro- and Microdiversity from Pole to Pole," *Cell* 177, no. 5 (May 2019): 1109–1123.e14, doi: 10.1016/j.cell.2019.03.040. Epub 2019 Apr 25.

5 See Jonathan Lambert, "Scientists Discover Nearly 200,000 Kinds of Ocean Viruses," *Abstractions* (blog), *Quanta Magazine,* April 25, 2019, https://www.quantamagazine.org/scientists-discover-nearly-200000-kinds-of-ocean-viruses-20190425/.

6 See Nathan Wolfe, "What's Left to Explore?" TED2012, https://www.ted.com/talks/nathan_wolfe_what_s_left_to_explore/transcript?language=en. Also see his book *The Viral Storm: The Dawn of a New Pandemic Age* (New York: Times Books, 2011).

7 See Evan Ratliff, "We Can Protect the Economy from Pandemics. Why Didn't We?" *Wired,* June 16, 2020, https://www

.wired.com/story/nathan-wolfe-global-economic-fallout-pandemic-insurance/.

8 See Neeraja Sankaran, "On the Historical Significance of Beijerinck and His Contagium Vivum Fluidum for Modern Virology," *History and Philosophy of the Life Sciences* 40, no. 3 (July 2018): 41, doi: 10 .1007/s40656-018-0206-1.

9 For a review of Koch's postulates, see the entry "Koch's postulates" at ScienceDirect.com, https://www.sciencedirect.com/topics/medicine-and-dentistry/kochs-postulates.

10 See Stanley's entry at the Nobel Prize organization's website at https://www .nobelprize.org/prizes/chemistry/1946/stanley/facts/.

11 See Theresa Machemer, "How a Few Sick Tobacco Plants Led Scientists to Unravel the Truth About Viruses," *Smithsonian Magazine,* March 24, 2020, https:// www.smithsonianmag.com/science-nature/what-are-viruses-history-tobacco-mosaic-disease-180974480/.

12 For everything you want to know about the genetic codes to life, see Walter Isaacson's book *The Code Breaker: Jennifer Doudna, Gene Editing, and the Future of the Human Race* (New York: Simon &

Schuster, 2021).

13 See *Coronaviruses: Are They Here to Stay?* News report from the United Nations Environment Program, April 3, 2020, https://www.unep.org/news-and-stories/story/coronaviruses-are-they-here-stay. Also access the UN's *Frontiers 2016 Report: Emerging Issues of Environmental Concern* at https://environmentlive.unep.org/media/docs/assessments/UNEP_Frontiers_2016_report_emerging_issues_of_environmental_concern.pdf.

14 The Centers for Disease Control and Prevention keeps records of these events on its site at www.cdc.gov.

15 See Vikram Misra, "Bats and Viruses," *Lancet Infectious Diseases* 20, no. 12 (December 2020): P1380, doi: 10.1016/S1473-3099(20)30743-X.

16 Numerous studies and articles have been published on the history and nature of coronaviruses. For an easy read see David Cyranoski, "Profile of a Killer: The Complex Biology Powering the Coronavirus Pandemic," *Nature* 581 (2020): 22–26, https://www.nature.com/articles/d41586-020-01315-7, doi: 10.1038/d41586-020-01315-7.

17 See James W. LeDuc and M. Anita Barry, "SARS, the First Pandemic of the 21st

Century," *Emerging Infectious Diseases* 10, no. 11 (November 2004): e26, doi: 10.3201/eid1011.040797_02.

18 See Matthew Pottinger, "Return of SARS Sparks Concerns About Lab Safety," *Wall Street Journal,* April 26, 2004, https://www.wsj.com/articles/SB10 82882396869992644.

19 See https://jamiemetzl.com/.

20 See Ben Hu et al., "Discovery of a Rich Gene Pool of Bat SARS-related Coronaviruses Provides New Insights into the Origin of SARS Coronavirus," *PLoS Pathogens* 13, no. 11 (November 2017): e1006698, doi: 10.1371/journal.ppat .1006698. Also see V. Menachery et al., "A SARS-like Cluster of Circulating Bat Coronaviruses Shows Potential for Human Emergence," *Nature Medicine* 21 (2015): 1508–1513, doi: 10.1038/nm .3985.

21 See Shi Zhengli et al., "Bat Coronaviruses in China," *Viruses* 11, no. 3 (March 2019): 210, doi: 10.3390/v11030210. Also see Jie Cui, Fang Li, and Shi Zhengli, "Origin and Evolution of Pathogenic Coronaviruses," *Nature Reviews Microbiology* 17 (2019): 181–192, doi: 10.1038/ s41579-018-0118-9.

22 Hu et al., "Discovery of a Rich Gene

Pool of Bat SARS-related Coronaviruses Provides New Insights into the Origin of SARS Coronavirus."

23 See Shi Zhengli et al., "Hantavirus Outbreak Associated with Laboratory Rats in Yunnan, China," *Infection, Genetics and Evolution* 10, no. 5 (July 2010): 638–644, doi: 10.1016/j.meegid.2010.03.015. Epub 2010 Apr 7.

24 See Jane Qiu, "How China's 'Bat Woman' Hunted Down Viruses from SARS to the New Coronavirus," *Scientific American,* June 1, 2020, https://www .scientificamerican.com/article/how-chinas-bat-woman-hunted-down-viruses-from-sars-to-the-new-coronavirus1/.

25 See Lesley Stahl's interview with Jamie Metzl, "What Happened in Wuhan? Why Questions Still Linger on the Origin of the Coronavirus," *60 Minutes,* March 28, 2021, https://www.cbsnews.com/news/ covid-19-wuhan-origins-60-minutes-2021-03-28/.

26 Alan Burdick, "Monster or Machine? A Profile of the Coronavirus at 6 Months," *New York Times,* June 2, 2020, https:// www.nytimes.com/ 2020/06/02/health/ coronavirus-profile-covid.html.

27 Ibid.

28 Ibid.

29 See Ahmed O. Kaseb et al., "The Impact of Angiotensin-Converting Enzyme 2 (ACE2) Expression on the Incidence and Severity of COVID-19 Infection," *Pathogens* 10, no. 3 (March 2021): 379, doi: 10.3390/path ogens10030379.

30 See James A. Robb and Clifford W. Bond, "Coronaviridae," in *Comprehensive Virology,* ed. Heinz Fraenkel-Conrat and Robert R. Wagner, vol. 14 (New York: Springer, 1979).

31 See Sasha Peiris et al., "Pathological Findings in Organs and Tissues of Patients with COVID-19: A Systematic Review," *PLoS One* 16, no. 4 (April 2021): e0250708, doi: 10.1371/journal.pone .0250708.

32 See Bina Choi et al., "Persistence and Evolution of SARS-CoV-2 in an Immunocompromised Host," *New England Journal of Medicine* 383, no. 23 (December 2020): 2291–2293, doi: 10.1056/NEJ Mc2031364.

33 Ibid.

34 See Meredith Wadman et al., "How Does Coronavirus Kill? Clinicians Trace a Ferocious Rampage through the Body, from Brain to Toes," *Science,* April 17, 2020, https://www.sciencemag.org/news/2020/ 04/how-does-coronavirus-kill-clinicians-

trace-ferocious-rampage-through-body-brain-toes.

35 Ibid.

Chapter 4: Cows

1 Moderna keeps a timeline of their developments on their website at https://investors.modernatx.com/news-releases. Their data on the safety and efficacy of the vaccine were published in the *New England Journal of Medicine*: Lindsey R. Baden et al., "Efficacy and Safety of the mRNA-1273 SARS-CoV-2 Vaccine," *New England Journal of Medicine* 384, no. 5 (February 2021): 403–416, doi: 10.1056/NEJMoa2035389. Epub 2020 Dec 30.

2 See "Covid-19 Vaccines Have Alerted the World to the Power of RNA Therapies," *Economist,* May 27, 2021, https://www.economist.com/briefing/2021/03/27/covid-19-vaccines-have-alerted-the-world-to-the-power-of-rna-therapies.

3 You'll find the story of smallpox in a lot of places, and here's one: Stefan Riedel, "Edward Jenner and the History of Smallpox and Vaccination," *Baylor University Medical Center Proceedings* 18, no. 1 (January 2005): 21–25, doi: 10.1080/08998280.2005.11928028.

4 See Livia Schrick et al., "An Early American Smallpox Vaccine Based on Horsepox," *New England Journal of Medicine* 377, no. 15 (October 2017): 1491–1492. doi: 10.1056/NEJMc1707600.

5 See Larry Brilliant, *Sometimes Brilliant: The Impossible Adventure of a Spiritual Seeker and Visionary Physician Who Helped Conquer the Worst Disease in History* (San Francisco: Harper One, 2016).

6 See Steven Johnson, *Extra Life: A Short History of Living Longer* (New York: Riverhead, 2021).

7 See Miles Parks, "Few Facts, Millions of Clicks: Fearmongering Vaccine Stories Go Viral Online," NPR, March 25, 2021, https://www.npr.org/2021/03/25/980035707/lying-through-truth-misleading-facts-fuel-vaccine-misinformation. Also see cdc.gov and weather.gov/safety/lightning-odds.

8 For a comprehensive history of the anti-vaccine movement, see the History of Vaccines website by the College of Physicians of Philadelphia at https://www.historyofvaccines.org/content/articles/history-anti-vaccination-movements.

9 See Peter Hotez, *Preventing the Next Pandemic: Vaccine Diplomacy in a Time of Anti-science* (Baltimore: Johns Hopkins

University Press, 2021).

10 For a basic understanding of vaccine technology, including how the new COVID vaccines work, see cdc.gov.

11 See Anthony Komaroff, MD, "Why Are mRNA Vaccines so Exciting?" *Harvard Health Blog,* December 10, 2020, https://www.health.harvard.edu/blog/why-are-mrna-vaccines-so-exciting-2020121021 599.

12 For a short version of the long story, see Diana Kwon, "The Promise of mRNA Vaccines," *Scientist,* November 25, 2020, https://www.the-scientist.com/news-opinion/the-promise-of-mrna-vaccines-68202.

13 See David Cox, "How mRNA Went from a Scientific Backwater to a Pandemic Crusher," *Wired,* December 2, 2020, https://www.wired.co.uk/article/mrna-coronavirus-vaccine-pfizer-biontech.

14 See Sanjay Gupta and Andrea Kane, "Do Some People Have Protection Against the Coronavirus?" CNN, August 2, 2020, https://www.cnn.com/2020/08/02/health/gupta-coronavirus-t-cell-cross-reactivity-immunity-wellness/index.html.

15 Thaddeus Stappenbeck, "If You Don't Get Sick After Your COVID-19 Vaccination, Does It Mean Your Immune System

Isn't Working?" Cleveland Clinic, "Health Essentials." February 16, 2021, https://health.clevelandclinic.org/if-you-dont-get-sick-after-your-covid-19-vaccination-does-it-mean-your-immune-system-isnt-working/.

16 See Amanda Sealy, "Manufacturing Moonshot: How Pfizer Makes Its Millions of Covid-19 Vaccine Doses," CNN, April 2, 2021, https://www.cnn.com/2021/03/31/health/pfizer-vaccine-manufacturing/index.html.

17 See Dr. Sanjay Gupta, "Benefits of Vaccines Are a Matter of Fact," CNN, January 10, 2017, https://www.cnn.com/2017/01/10/health/vaccines-sanjay-gupta/index.html.

18 Several credible sites have debunked myths about the COVID vaccines and continue to post updates. Among them: Johns Hopkins Medicine at https://www.hopkinsmedicine.org/health/conditions-and-diseases/coronavirus/covid-19-vaccines-myth-versus-fact; and the American Association of American Medical Colleges (AAMC) at https://www.aamc.org/news-insights/6-myths-about-covid-19-vaccines-debunked.

19 See Brenda Goodman, "Why Covid Vaccines Are Falsely Linked to Infertility,"

WebMD, January 12, 2021, https://www
.webmd.com/vaccines/covid-19-vaccine/
news/20210112/why-covid-vaccines-are-
falsely-linked-to-infertility.

20 See Sarah Zhang, "The Oldest Virus
Ever Sequenced Comes from a 7,000-
Year-Old Tooth," *Atlantic,* May 9, 2018,
https://www.theatlantic.com/science/
archive/2018/05/a-7000-year-old-virus-
sequenced-from-a-neolithic-mans-tooth/
559862/.

21 See Matthieu Legendre et al., "In-depth
Study of Mollivirus sibericum, a New
30,000-y-old Giant Virus Infecting Acan-
thamoeba," *Proceedings of the National
Academy of Sciences of the USA* 112, no.
38 (September 2015): E5327–335, doi:
10.1073/pnas.1510795112. Epub 2015
Sep 8.

Chapter 5: P: Plan Ahead

1 See Bonnie Henry, *Be Kind, Be Calm, Be
Safe: Four Weeks that Shaped a Pandemic*
(Toronto: Penguin Canada, 2021).

2 See Catherine Porter, "The Top Doctor
Who Aced the Coronavirus Test," *New
York Times,* June 5, 2020, https://www
.nytimes.com/2020/06/05/world/canada/
bonnie-henry-british-columbia-coronavi

rus.html.

3 See Thom Barker, "Dr. Bonnie Henry Given New Name in B.C. First Nation Ceremony: 'One Who Is Calm among Us'," Victoria News, May 26, 2020, https://www.vicnews.com/news/dr-bonnie-henry-given-new-name-in-b-c-first-nations-ceremony-one-who-is-calm-among-us/.

4 See Nicholas A. Christakis, *Apollo's Arrow: The Profound and Enduring Impact of Coronavirus on the Way We Live* (New York: Little, Brown Spark, 2020).

5 See Albert Camus, *The Plague,* trans. Stuart Gilbert (New York: Knopf, 1948).

6 See Metabiota.com.

7 See Ben Oppenheim et al., "Assessing Global Preparedness for the Next Pandemic: Development and Application of an Epidemic Preparedness Index," *BMJ Global Health* 4 (2019): e001157, https://gh.bmj.com/content/4/1/e001157. Also see Evan Ratliff, "We Can Protect the Economy from Pandemics. Why Didn't We?" *Wired,* June 16, 2020, https://www.wired.com/story/nathan-wolfe-global-economic-fallout-pandemic-insurance/.

8 See Dean T. Jamison et al., *Disease Control Priorities,* 3rd ed., vol. 9, *Improving Health and Reducing Poverty* (Washington,

DC: World Bank, 2017), https://open knowledge.worldbank.org/handle/10986/28877.

9 See Jin Pan et al., "Inward and Outward Effectiveness of Cloth Masks, a Surgical Mask, and a Face Shield," *Aerosol Science and Technology* 55, no. 6 (2021): 718–733, doi: 10.1080/02786826.2021.1890687.

10 See Jennifer Prah Ruger, "The CDC Is a National Treasure. Why Is It Being Sidelined?" CNN, "Opinion," May 15, 2020, https://www.cnn.com/2020/05/14/opinions/pandemic-amnesia-threatens-our-health-cdc-prah-ruger/index.html.

11 See the report "A Funding Crisis for Public Health and Safety," by Trust for America's Health at https://www.tfah.org/report-details/a-funding-crisis-for-public-health-and-safety-state-by-state-and-federal-public-health-funding-facts-and-recommendations/.

12 See Jason Kottke, "The Paradox of Preparation," *kottke.org* (blog), March 16, 2020, https://kottke.org/20/03/the-paradox-of-preparation.

Chapter 6: R: Rethink and Rewire Risk in Your Brain

1 This quote is attributed to James D. Watson and is written in the foreword to Sandra Ackerman's *Discovering the Brain* (Washington, DC: National Academies Press, 1992).
2 E. Awad et al., "The Moral Machine Experiment," *Nature* 563 (2018): 59–64, doi: 10.1038/s41586-018-0637-6. Also see https://www.moral machine.net/.
3 To access all of Shohamy's work and studies, go to https://shohamylab.zuckerman institute .columbia.edu/ research-projects. Also see https://zuckermaninstitute .columbia.edu/daphna-shohamy-phd.
4 See https://www.idsociety.org/.
5 See Martin Z. Bazant and John W. M. Bush, "A Guideline to Limit Indoor Airborne Transmission of COVID-19," *Proceedings of the National Academy of Sciences of the USA* 118, no. 17 (April 2021): e2018995118, doi: 10.1073/pnas.201899 5118.
6 See Kathy Katella, "The Johnson & Johnson Vaccine and Blood Clots: What You Need to Know," Yale Medicine, April 23, 2021, https://www.yalemedicine.org/ news/coronavirus-vaccine-blood-clots.

7 See cdc.gov.

8 See Maggie Fox, "These Blood Clot Experts Want You to Get a Covid-19 Vaccine. Here's Why," CNN, April 21, 2021, https://www.cnn.com/2021/04/20/health/blood-clots-experts-covid-vaccine/index.html.

9 For a basic lesson on risk, with examples, see "Understanding Risk," BMJ Best Practice site at https://stg-bestpractice.bmj.com/info/toolkit/practise-ebm/understanding-risk/.

10 See Andrea Kane, "These Twins Were Like Two Peas in a Pod — Except When Covid-19 Struck," CNN, May 8, 2021, https://www.cnn.com/2021/05/08/health/identical-twins-covid-19-severe-illness/index.html.

11 See "The Disinformation Dozen" by the Center for Countering Digital Hate, March 24, 2021, https://252f2edd-1c8b-49f5-9bb2-cb57bb47e4ba.filesusr.com/ugd/f4d9b9_b7cedc0553604720b7137f8663366ee5.pdf. Also see Shannon Bond, "Just 12 People Are Behind Most Vaccine Hoaxes on Social Media, Research Shows," NPR, May 14, 2021, https://www.npr.org/2021/05/13/996570855/disinformation-dozen-test-facebooks-twitters-ability-to-curb-vaccine-hoaxes.

12 Michael Eisenstein, "What's Your Risk of Catching COVID? These Tools Help You to Find Out," *Nature* 589 (December 2021): 158–159.

13 See David Leonhardt, "What Do You Do When the Kids Are Still Unvaccinated?" *New York Times,* April 22, 2021, https://www.nytimes.com/2021/04/22/opinion/covid-vaccine-kids.html.

Chapter 7: O: Optimize Health

1 See Alaa Elassar, "He Was an Athlete in the Best Shape of His Life. Then Covid-19 Nearly Killed Him," CNN, June 30, 2020, https://www.cnn.com/2020/06/30/health/coronavirus-athlete-covid-19-ahmad-ayyad-johns-hopkins-trnd/index.html.

2 See Elian Peltier and Vanessa Friedman, "Alber Elbaz, Beloved Fashion Designer, Is Dead at 59," Obituaries, *New York Times,* April 25, 2021, https://www.nytimes.com/2021/04/25/obituaries/alber-elbaz-dead.html.

3 See the International Food Information Council's 2020 Food and Health Survey at https://foodinsight.org/wp-content/uploads/2020/06/ IFIC-Food-and-Health-Survey-2020.pdf.

4 See "Blue Cross Blue Shield Association

Study Finds Millennials Are Less Healthy than Generation X Were at the Same Age," Blue Cross Blue Shield, April 24, 2019, https://www.bcbs.com/press-releases/blue-cross-blue-shield-association-study-finds-millennials-are-less-healthy. Also see Megan Leonhardt, "44% of Older Millennials Already Have a Chronic Health Condition. Here's What that Means for Their Futures," CNBC, May 4, 2019, https://www.cnbc.com/2021/05/04/older-millennials-chronic-health-conditions.html.

5 See cdc.gov.

6 See Meredith Wadman, "Why COVID-19 Is More Deadly in People with Obesity — Even If They're Young," *Science,* September 8, 2020, https://www.sciencemag.org/news/2020/09/why-covid-19-more-deadly-people-obesity-even-if-theyre-young.

7 See Manfred J Müller, Anja Bosy-Westphal, and Steven B. Heymsfield, "Is There Evidence for a Set Point that Regulates Human Body Weight?" *Faculty of 1000 Medicine Reports* 2 (August 2010): 59, doi: 10.3410/M2-59.

8 See cdc.gov.

9 See "Dietary Supplements in the Time of COVID-19" at NIH.gov, https://ods.nih.gov/factsheets/COVID19-HealthPro

fessional/, and "FDA and the Federal Trade Commission (FTC) Sent 106 Joint Warning Letters to Supplement Producers for Selling Products" at ftc.gov, https://www.ftc.gov/news-events/press-releases/2021/05/federal-trade-commission-fda-warn-five-companies-may-be-illegally.

10 For everything you want to know about the microbiome, I recommend: Liam Drew, "Highlights from Studies on the Gut Microbiome," *Nature* 577 (2020): S24–25, https://www.nature.com/articles/d41586-020-00203-4. Also see Emeran Mayer, *The Mind-Gut Connection: How the Hidden Conversation Within Our Bodies Impacts Our Mood, Our Choices, and Our Overall Health* (New York: Harper Wave, 2016).

11 See H. F. Helander and L. Fändriks, "Surface Area of the Digestive Tract — Revisited," *Scandinavian Journal of Gastroenterology* 49, no. 6 (June 2014): 681–89, doi: 10.3109/00365521.2014.898326.

12 See Y. K. Yeoh et al., "Gut Microbiota Composition Reflects Disease Severity and Dysfunctional Immune Responses in Patients with COVID-19," *Gut* 70 (2021): 698–706, doi: 10.1136/gutjnl-2020-323020.

13 See cdc.gov.

14 See L. Laranjo et al., "Do Smartphone Applications and Activity Trackers Increase Physical Activity in Adults? Systematic Review, Meta-analysis and Metaregression," *British Journal of Sports Medicine* 55 (2021): 422–432, doi: 10.1136/bjsports-2020-102892.

15 For everything you want to know about sleep, see: Matthew Walker, *Why We Sleep: Unlocking the Power of Sleep and Dreams* (New York: Scribner, 2017).

16 For a general overview, see Suzanne C. Segerstrom and Gregory E. Miller, "Psychological Stress and the Human Immune System: A Meta-analytic Study of 30 Years of Inquiry," *Psychological Bulletin Journal* 130, no. 4 (July 2004): 601–630, doi: 10.1037/00332909.130.4.601.

17 See Richard A. Friedman, "You Might Be Depressed Now, but Don't Underestimate Your Resilience," *New York Times,* May 4, 2021.

18 See Chris Melore, "Lonely Nation: 2 in 3 Americans Feel More Alone than Ever Before, Many Admit to Crying for First Time in Years," Study Finds, April 29, 2021, https://www.studyfinds.org/lonely-nation-two-thirds-feel-more-alone-than-ever-many-cry-first-time/.

19 See Roger A. H. Adan et al., "Nutritional

Psychiatry: Towards Improving Mental Health by What You Eat," *European Neuropsychopharmacology* 29, no. 12 (December 2019): 1321–1332, doi: 10.1016/j.euroneuro.2019.10.011.

20 See Felice N. Jacka, "Nutritional Psychiatry: Where to Next?" *EBio-Medicine* 17 (March 2017): 24–29, doi: 10.1016/j.ebiom.2017.02.020.

Chapter 8: O: Organize Family

1 See Sanjay Gupta, *Childhood, Interrupted: Raising Kids During a Pandemic,* Audible Originals (2020).

2 See "What Have Scientists Learned about Kids' Well-being from Pandemic?" *Full Circle,* CNN, April 1, 2021, https://www.cnn.com/videos/health/2021/04/01/angela-duckworth-grit-help-kids-thrive-pandemic-full-episode-acfc-vpx.cnn.

3 See Phil McCausland, "Medical Debt Is Engulfing More People as Pandemic Takes Its Toll," NBC News, April 23, 2021, https://www.nbcnews.com/politics/politics-news/medical-debt-engulfing-more-people-pandemic-takes-its-toll-n1265002.

4 See "About 8% of People Who Live in US Long-term-care Facilities Have Died of COVID-19 — Nearly 1 in 12. For

Nursing Homes Alone, the Figure Is Nearly 1 in 10," The Covid Tracking Project, https://covidtracking.com/nursing-homes-long-term-care-facilities.

5 See "Infection Control Deficiencies Were Widespread and Persistent in Nursing Homes Prior to COVID-19 Pandemic," Report by the US Government Accountability Office, May 20, 2020, https://www.gao.gov/products/gao-20-576r.

6 See Kim Schive, "Public Toilets and 'Toilet Plumes'," MIT Medical, June 15, 2020, https://medical.mit.edu/covid-19-updates/2020/06/public-toilets-and-toilet-plumes.

7 See D. P. Strachan, "Hay Fever, Hygiene, and Household Size," *British Medical Journal* 299, no. 6710 (November 1989): 1259–1260, doi: 10.1136/bmj.299.6710.1259.

8 See Linda Brookes and Laurence E. Cheng, "The Hygiene Hypothesis — Redefine, Rename, or Just Clean It Up?" Medscape, April 6, 2015, https://www.medscape.com/viewarticle/842500.

9 B. Brett Finlay et al., "The Hygiene Hypothesis, the COVID Pandemic, and Consequences for the Human Microbiome," *Proceedings of the National Academy of Sciences* 118, no. 6 (February 2021):

e2010217118, doi: 10.1073/pnas.2010 217118.

10 See S. Lopez-Leon et al., "More than 50 Long-term Effects of COVID-19: A Systematic Review and Meta-analysis," preprint, *medRxiv,* posted January 30, 2021, doi: 10.1101/2021.01.27.21250617. Also see Judy George, "80% of COVID-19 Patients May Have Lingering Symptoms, Signs — More than 50 Effects Persisted After Acute Infection, Meta-analysis Shows," MedPage Today, January 30, 2021, https://www.medpagetoday.com/ infectiousdisease/covid19/90966.

11 See "Gene Expression Changes Could Be Behind Long-Haul COVID-19 Symptoms," Clinical Omics, April 27, 2021, https://www.clinicalomics.com/topics/ patient-care/coronavirus/gene-expression-changes-could-be-behind-long-haul-covid-19-symptoms/.

12 See cdc.gov.

13 See https://www.survivorcorps.com/.

Chapter 9: F: Fight for the Future of Us

1 See Dr. Sanjay Gupta, "I Went to Afghanistan and All I Got Was H1N1," CNN, September 23, 2009.

2 See cdc.gov.

3 See Josh Holder, "Tracking Coronavirus Vaccinations Around the World," *New York Times,* June 4, 2021, https://www.nytimes.com/interactive/2021/world/covid-vaccinations-tracker.html.

4 See E. Dong, H. Du, and L. Gardner, "An Interactive Web-based Dashboard to Track COVID-19 in Real Time," *Lancet Infectious Diseases* 20 no. 5 (2020): 533–534, doi: 10.1016/S1473-3099(20)30120-1. Also see https://www.github.com/CSSEGISandData/COVID-19.

5 Ibid.

6 See Jeffrey Gettleman, Shalini Venugopal, and Apoorva Mandavilli, "India Blames a Virus Variant as Its Covid-19 Crisis Deepens," *New York Times,* April 28, 2021, https://www.nytimes.com/2021/04/28/world/asia/india-covid19-variant.html.

7 See Christopher Klein, "Why October 1918 Was America's Deadliest Month Ever," History, October 5, 2018, https://www.history.com/news/spanish-flu-deaths-october-1918.

8 See Grace Hauck, "We're Celebrating Thanksgiving Amid a Pandemic. Here's How We Did It in 1918 — and What Happened Next," *USA Today,* November 21, 2020, https://www.usatoday.com/in-depth/news/nation/2020/11/21/covid-and-

thanksgiving-how-we-celebrated-during-1918-flu-pandemic/6264231002/.

ABOUT THE AUTHOR

Sanjay Gupta grew up in a small midwestern town, married his college sweetheart, and can now be found getting mercilessly teased by his three teenage daughters. When not receiving unsolicited fashion advice from them, he spends his time as an associate chief of neurosurgery, bestselling author, and award-winning television correspondent. He is a member of the National Academy of Medicine and the Academy of Arts and Sciences. He is particularly proud of his as yet undiscovered shower singing voice and is currently on a hunt for the world's most perfect nap.

The employees of Thorndike Press hope you have enjoyed this Large Print book. All our Thorndike, Wheeler, and Kennebec Large Print titles are designed for easy reading, and all our books are made to last. Other Thorndike Press Large Print books are available at your library, through selected bookstores, or directly from us.

For information about titles, please call:
   (800) 223-1244

or visit our website at:
   gale.com/thorndike

To share your comments, please write:
   Publisher
   Thorndike Press
   10 Water St., Suite 310
   Waterville, ME 04901